Saul Bellow Journal

| Volume 7 | Number 1 | Winter 1988 |

Contents

Articles

Book Reviews

Move Over, Menander. Bellow Has Gone from New Comedy to the Sublime

Dolly Smith
University of Texas at Tyler

At the very end of *The Last Analysis*, Bummy is ready for the sublime, a new New Comedy which differs from the old New Comedy of Menander. Nearly 2,300 years separate Menander—the leading writer of New Comedy—and Saul Bellow. In all that time surprisingly little has been written that would structurally alter the dramatic comedy style that Menander developed in ancient Greece. Gilbert Murray notes that ancient critics looked on Menander's art as the "very summit of naturalness and closeness to life," viewing him as they did "in contrast to both the wild extravagances of the Old Comedy and to the heroic legends and 'large utterance' which formed the theme and method of tragedy" (7). Menander's comedies were sacred plays, written to be performed at the festival of Dionysus (8) and as such celebrated the "annual discovery, when all the earth seems dead, of that Renewal of Life [now thought of as] the New Year of Spring" (120).

Menander includes in his comedies either a "mysterious foundling baby" or a "pregnant heroine who bears a child to an unknown or secret father" (8). The baby's "recognition" lifts him "to wealth and fortune" (121). The characters with whom Menander peopled his comedies are "ordinary men and women, not divine nor heroic nor even royal" (7). As to how an artist of Menander's obvious genius could be content to write play after play with the same stock characters and predictable action and outcome of plot, Murray notes that "the workings of tradition in all art . . . are extremely subtle." He adds, "We merely do without question the thing we are in the habit of doing. Consciousness comes in when there is some clash between the tradition and the artist's own desires" (9–10). It is possible just such a clash between tradition and desire took place within Saul Bellow, and the result of that clash was *The Last Analysis* and the new comic theory advanced in it by Bummidge—the theory of Sublime Comedy.

As the play opens, Bummy has come to the realization that people are laughing at all the wrong things. In an attempt to help people come to know themselves—and thus understand why they laugh—Bummy wants to bring his "*Existenz*-Action-Self-analysis" to the public. His cousin Winkleman accuses him of being a " 'mental climber' " and reminds him that he is a " 'comic not a scientist' " (674), but Bummy is not daunted. Throughout the play runs an on-going, informal, sub-surface survey of laughter: how people laugh, when and why they laugh (or fail to laugh), and how this laughter serves them and/or affects others.

Taunted by Winkleman that he has " 'lost his touch,' " Bummy responds that he can still make " 'those apes laugh any time. At will.' " However, he can no longer stand the sound they make when they laugh (676). Bummy recounts the dream he dreamt the night before and—while describing the monster he saw—Bummy remembers, " 'He/she was laughing. . . . He-he-he! Ha! Hoo-hoo-hoo! That laughter! Now I'm afraid I may not be taken seriously in the field of science. And I no longer know what laughter is' " (679). In response to Bummy's questioning the pass he just made at Imogen, the Technician just laughs. Bummy is angered and says, " 'Listen to that laugh. Is that neurotic or is that neurotic? Boy, what decadence! Malignancy in the marrow of society' " (679). When Bummy's sister Madge arrives, he tells her he needs five thousand dollars. Madge laughs. Bellow's stage directions say that Bummy "behaves oddly when she laughs; puts ear to her chest like a physician" and asks her, " 'That makes you laugh? Laugh again.' " Bummy tells Madge, " 'Your laughter fascinates me. Mama had a throaty laugh. Yours has little screams and cries in it.' " Bummy then imitates Madge's laugh (681).

Bummy [the patient] tells Bummy [the analyst] about his father's rejection, even after Bummy had become a success:

> "The good-for-nothing became a star and earned millions making people laugh—all but Papa. He never laughed. . . . Laugh, you old Turk. Never! Censure. . . . But Bummidge is still spilling gravy at life's banquet and out front they're laughing fit to bust." (He laughs, closer to tears.) "Yes, I am that crass man, Bummidge. Oh, how foul my soul is! I have the Pagliacce Gangrene. Ha, ha, ha—weep, weep, weep!" (687)

Then Bummy remembers his mother: " 'She laughed. Oh what a fat throaty laugh she had. Her apron shook' " (687).

His son Max questions Bummy's analysis by asking, " 'What makes a comic think he can cure human perversity?' " Bummy, insulted, responds that while he is " '*only* a comic' " he still " 'knows what he knows.' " He tells Max that " 'audiences laughing' " look " 'monstrous' " from the stage: " 'Oh, the despair, my son! The stale hearts! The snarling and gasping!' " Bummy is then directed to imitate the audience "snarling, savage, frightening, howling, quavering" as he says: " 'Ha ha—I am a cow, a sheep, a wolf, a rat. I am a victim, a killer. Ha, ha—my soul is corked forever. Let me out. My spirit is famished. I twist and rub. Ha, ha, ha, I'm an imposter. . . . Life has no meaning. Ha, ha, ha, ha, ha!' " (691). When his wife, Bella, warns Bummy that the intellectuals will laugh at him, he responds, " 'They know nothing about laughing. That's my field' " (702). Demonstrating—with the help of the rest of the cast—what life was like at the height of his career as a comic, Bummy recalls, " 'People laugh at everything I say. "Nice day." ' (To group.) 'Laugh!' (They laugh uproariously.) 'You see how it worked. "Nice day." ' (They laugh again. He sneezes.)" (716).

Just before he is overcome by an attack of " 'Humanitis—an emotional disorder of our relation to the human condition [during which] being human is too much' " (714), Bummy explains his original decision to become a comedian: " 'I chose to serve laughter, but the weight of suffering overcame me time and again' " (724).

Finally, as Bummy prepares to " 'die to the old corn,' " he bids " 'farewell to the old jokes' " and—crawling into a wardrobe basket—states:

> "The dark night of my soul has begun. . . . I die of banality. Lay me in this mirthless tomb, and cover me with corn. Let me hear the laughter of evil for the last time. Oh, demons who murder while guffawing, I have succumbed. . . . Consummatum est. It is ended." (726)

But Bummy is not dead. Like Menander, Bellow's comedy also celebrates the renewal of life. Bummy is summoned forth from his "tomb" and is reborn. Imogen calls, " 'Come forth, Lazarus' " and Bummy arises (762). Into what kind of world is he reborn? A world where Bella and Max, Madge and Winkleman, Pamela and Fiddleman are all waiting to hitch their wagons to Bummy's new star. Bummy's "comic method" had begun only after his " 'self got lost' " (694). He had been " 'exploited' " and " 'dragged down into affluence,' " changing his name and leading a false life (676). And this is exactly what his family and old associates want from him again. Fiddleman, the impresario, has rushed over—with police escort—from the Waldorf to wave a handful of option checks under Bummy's nose (735). Pamela, who up to now has found her life as Bummy's paramour a pretense and a " 'drag' " (695), looks ahead: " 'No more living in filth. What a future lies before us!' " (732). Madge and Winkleman, who at first denounce Bummy's theories as " 'insane' " and his mind as " 'twisted,' " quickly reverse their opinions upon hearing of the success of his broadcast and realize that they might in fact have a chance to remain untouched by the nursing home scandal (731). Max, who had been ready to stop Bummy's broadcast with a restraining order (706), suddenly develops a feeling of deep kinship with his father: " 'We've got business. Keep 'em [the scientists] out. Let the family settle first' " (732). Bella—having learned that Bummy has " 'attained rebirth' " but is uncertain as to just who he is—promises: " 'We'll tell you. We'll straighten you out. Don't worry, kid' " (733). She sees in Bummy's "rebirth" another chance at realizing her dream of being " 'the greatest family in America, on the cover of *Time*' " (731).

But this is not new life at all. It is a life full of the same tired jokes and the same pointless laughter which Bummy "died" to escape. When his family and the old hangers-on refuse to leave, Bellow's directions state that a device is lowered from above (736). All but Bummy, Imogen, and Bertram are caught in a net and dragged off stage. Donning his toga, Bummy prepares to meet with his scientific colleagues. He has passed through the " 'brutal stage of life' " and the " 'mediocre stage.' " He is now ready for the " 'sublime' " (737).

The sublime, as discussed by Longinus in his treatise *On the Sublime*, is a "thing of spirit," a "spark leaping from writer to reader," not a "product of technique." Edmund Burke's theory of the sublime is that a "painful idea creates a sublime passion." By doing so, it "concentrate[s] the mind on that single facet of experience" and produces a "momentary suspension of rational activity, uncertainty, and self-consciousness" (Holman 433).

Bellow's choice of the word *sublime* indicates a translation of Burke's theory from the tragic to the comic. The sublime would be a joyful thought or idea that creates a sublime passion that holds the concentration of the mind, creating what Henri Bergson termed a "momentary anesthesia of the heart," an "absence of feeling" that allows the mind to put aside feelings of pity or affection in order to appreciate the comic aspect of any given situation (746).

What are the elements of Sublime Comedy? From the script of *The Last Analysis* come six points:

1. Comedy is the theater of the soul (730). The soul laughs, not the brain. The soul houses the comic spirit.

2. Comedy is not for intellectuals, who do not know how to laugh. Comedy is for the people of the streets (702).

3. Comedy celebrates love but does not make a production of it (702). Comedy allows love to happen. If love masks other emotions—greed or lust in particular—it is dishonest. " 'Wouldn't it be better to have a rutting season? Once a year, but the real thing? When the willows turn yellow in March?' " (734).

4. Comedy is salvation from tragedy, a method to evade suffering. " 'The forms—the many forms that suffering takes. The compulsion to suffer. But for each and every one of these there is method to evade suffering. Delusion. Intoxication. Ecstacy. And comedy' " (710–11).

5. The weakness of comedy is that " 'when the laughing stops, there's still a big surplus of pain.' " This pain is caused by "Pagliacci Gangrene," which is in turn caused " 'by failure of circulation. Cut off by self-pity. Passivity. Fear. Masochistic rage.' " "Pagliacci Gangrene" is " 'crying as you laugh, but making a fortune meanwhile' " (714–16). The solution?

6. Recover wit (725). Get rid of the old jokes (726). Reveal emotional truths, but in an absurd form (730). Launch a new search for humanhood:

> "To disown the individual altogether is nihilism, which isn't funny at all. But suppose all we fumblers and bumblers, we cranks and creeps and cripples, we proud, sniffling, ragged-assed paupers of heart and soul, sick with every personal vice, rattled, proud, spoiled, and distracted—suppose we look again for the manhood we are born to inherit." (726)

The result would be Sublime Comedy.

Unfortunately, what makes wonderful sense in theory did not exactly work out in fact. Of an opinion that seems to differ with Point Six is Robert R. Dutton, who faults *The Last Analysis* in several areas. It is his opinion that the play is "heavy with farcical elements that simply get out of hand." He also feels that "the stage is quite often entirely too busy, in an uproar most of the time." He finds Bellow's characters neither strong nor sympathetic, and he criticizes Bummy for losing the audience through his "slapstick behavior." Dutton ends his critique by stating, "It is not a good play, not a good comedy—except for those of us who delight in Bellow's mind in whatever form it is presented" (8). Also contrary to Point Six is Brigitte Scheer-Schäzler's opinion that one reason why the play fails is that Bellow tries to mix "comedy and seriousness." She notes the "seriousness mocks itself" but does so to a "degree of extent" difficult to determine. She states, "Bummidge's rebirth cannot be taken by the audience for what he himself takes it; if so, the playgoers could be accused of having missed the satire." However, she also finds that "Bummidge's aspirations are too great, the subject of the play too serious, to be treated only farcically" (114–15).

Bellow himself seems to contradict Points One and Two. Irving Malin quotes Bellow as having commented that the Broadway production of *The Last Analysis* "neglected" the "mental comedy" of his characters, and that the play's "real subject is the mind's comical struggle for survival in an environment of Ideas" (115), a concept closely linked to Henri Bergson's contention that the appeal of comedy is to "intelligence, pure and simple," and that this "intelligence . . . must always remain in touch with other intelligences" (746). In other words, in order for laughter to be understood, it must be put back into its "natural environment, which is society" (747). But society, the "people of the street," did not understand Bellow's Sublime Comedy. *The Last Analysis* closed after only 28 performances at the Belasco Theatre in 1964 (Dutton 8).

Why? Perhaps (quoting Winkleman on Bummy) Bellow " 'confused the Plain Man, and that's the sonofabitch that pays for the whole show ' " (678). Prior to his summary of the play in "Bummy's Analysis," Malin notes that he "read the text closely" (115), while Glenn M. Loney—in his headnote to *The Last Analysis*—says that the "flow of ideas, the variety of images, the fund of satire is all so rich that only reading—and rereading— can give the potential audience effective access to it" (670). Thus, both Malin and Loney also contradict the premises set forth in Points One and Two: that it is the soul—not the brain—that laughs, and that intellectuals do not know how to laugh. It is Loney's opinion that "Bellow writes for readers, not for viewers." Loney observes that it is "one thing to write a novel in dramatic form" but "quite another to write a playable play" and adds that much of *The Last Analysis* "has to be appreciated intellectually" (670). There is that word again—*intellectually*.

How did Bellow respond to the popular failure of *The Last Analysis*? He took the theory of Sublime Comedy and reworked the portions of Points One and Two that had proven themselves to be self-contradictory. He then applied them—along with the four remaining points—in a manner that left no doubt as to their validity: he wrote a novel entitled *Humboldt's Gift*. *Humboldt's Gift* not only proves the theory of Sublime Comedy through its plot as well as through the two movie scenarios which are a part of that plot, it also provides Bellow with a harmless personal revenge on all those playgoers who failed to appreciate *The Last Analysis*. The protagonist of *Humboldt's Gift* is Charlie Citrine, and Charlie is the author of a play entitled *Von Trenck* which ran as a hit at the Belasco Theatre for eight months before being made into an equally successful movie (15). How much of Bellow can be found in Charlie? Bellow was asked that question during the Southern Methodist University Literary Festival in 1976. As reported by Kent Biffle in a *Dallas Morning News* article entitled "Mr. Bellow's Planet," Bellow replied, "If anyone in any of my books needs something that I have, out of the kindness of my heart, I just lend it." To Charlie Citrine, Bellow lent his play-writing self, and to *Humboldt's Gift* he lent his theory of Sublime Comedy.

Bellow, in the process of reworking the troublesome areas of Points One and Two, shows how Charlie—who is himself considered an intellectual by others in the intellectual world—begins to pull away from that society. He moves from New York back to Chicago, to the dismay of his then-wife Denise, who defines his action as a "kind of mental suicide, death wish" (41). He begins seeing old friends such as George Swiebel again, but when he introduces George the "primitivist" to "intellectuals" such as his "learned friend Durnwald," the results are both disastrous and enlightening. The Swiebel/Durnwald incident clarifies that the problem with Points One and Two lies in the original wording's representing a contradiction of terms. Charlie realizes that "Humboldt, boyish, loved the life of the mind and I shared his enthusiasm. But the intellectuals one meets are something else again" (59). Therefore, Point One should read: Comedy *is* the theater of the soul, but it is the brain, the mind, the common sense, that first registers humor and then transmits the message to the soul. Logically, Point Two would then say: Comedy is *not* for the intellectuals who—in seeking still higher and higher levels of thought—have elevated themselves to an atmosphere so rarified that laughter can no longer exist. Comedy is for the intelligent people of the street. These people have gotten "out of the sensible world" and are now able to "feel parts of the soul awakening that had never been awake before"(223).

Intellectuals are "against the True, the Good, the Beautiful" (60). The scope of the intellectual has become too narrow: "The only art intellectuals can be interested in is an art which celebrates the primacy of ideas. . . . For them the whole purpose of art is to suggest and inspire ideas and discourse" (32). When he was young, Charlie believed that being an intellectual assured him of a "higher life," but now he thinks differently. He has decided to "listen to the voice of my own mind speaking from within, from my own depths." This voice tells him that "there was my body, in nature, and that there was also me" (186).

Once, inspired by a book lent him by Humboldt, Charlie had conceived a project that he hoped his daughter Mary would one day carry on after he himself has become "too old or too weak or too silly to continue." He still keeps notes and memos on the project for her, tucked away in a drawer. The project he had conceived was a "very personal overview of the Intellectual Comedy of the modern mind." Charlie comments that this would not be a "work of fiction but a different kind of imaginative projection" but does not elaborate any further on the topic (73).

Charlie eventually becomes "furious and arrogant and vengeful toward intellectuals" and asserts that they waste not only their own time but also that of everyone else and that he would like to "trample and clobber them" (356). Finally, in Spain, "elderly, heart injured, meditating in kitchen odors," Charlie realizes, "I had come to despise with all my heart" the "mental respectability of good members of educated society" (439).

Bellow's treatment of love in *Humboldt's Gift* again demonstrates Point Three: Comedy celebrates love, but it does not make a big production of it. Instead comedy allows love to happen. Charlie's first love was Naomi Lutz, but while he was away at college in Wisconsin "reading poetry and studying rotation pool at the Rathskeller," Naomi married a pawnbroker. Charlie later realizes that the financial security the other man could offer her was not the only reason for Naomi's decision; the "mental burdens and responsibilities of an intellectual's wife had frightened her" (76). Years later Charlie runs into Naomi in the bar of the hotel where he has come to attempt to seduce Renata for the first time and admits that he has often thought that because he had failed to marry Naomi, spend his life with her, hold her "in [his] arms nightly since the age of fifteen," he had lost his character (213). But he is not in the bar to renew old acquaintances; he is there to seduce Renata.

After Naomi's daughter Maggie bails Charlie out of jail (290), he goes to visit Naomi, a "sentimental visit" (296). Watching Naomi direct traffic at the school crossing, he thinks about this "woman for whom he once felt perfect love" (297). After brunch, they talk of love—past and present—and Charlie speaks of the only other girl he had ever truly loved: "Demmie Vonghel. Yes. She was the real thing, too" (300). Worried that Renata is using Charlie, Naomi tells him, " 'Don't wear yourself out proving something with these giant broads. Remember, your great love was for me, just five feet tall' " (308). In other words, do not make a big production of love; allow it to happen. But Charlie's affair has been a series of big productions from the beginning when his attempt to seduce Renata was foiled by too many martinis (217).

It was Renata who convinced him to buy the $18,000 Mercedes 280-SL (36). She had "forbidden [him] to drive a Dart," and when he tried to negotiate with the Mercedes salesman for a used model, "Renata—roused, florid, fragrant, large—had put her hand on the silver hood and said, 'This one—the coupe' " (44). Renata also encouraged Charlie to buy a "fancy check overcoat at Saks" (194), which Julius would later describe as "that horse blanket" (382). Both Charlie and Renata were guilty of making a big production of love; moreover, the love that they had for one another was dishonest, masking as it did all their hidden needs. It was in its own way as big a production as was the duplicate journey into paradise which Humboldt described in his *Treatment*: Corcoran reproduced the trip he and Laverne had taken—the second time taking his wife Hepzibah instead—so that he could publish a novel based on the first trip while still keeping his wife unaware of his infidelity (345). The venture was a failure; big productions often are.

However, there are other loves in *Humboldt's Gift* that the comedy does celebrate because they are honest and not contrived. Charlie genuinely loves Humboldt and Humboldt knows it (128). Charlie never loses his love for Humboldt—not when *Von Trenck* is picketed (159) and not when Humboldt cashes the "blood brother" check for $6,763 (130). Humboldt returns Charlie's love through his legacy to him. Humboldt leaves two movie scenarios that would eventually solve Charlie's money problems (482). More importantly, he bequeaths them jointly to Kathleen and Charlie in such a way that the two of them would be reunited (373).

Point Four states that comedy is salvation from tragedy, a method to evade suffering. Or, as Humboldt so succinctly puts it in his final letter to Charlie, "Prospero is a Hamlet who gets his revenge through art" (345). Point Four is aptly illustrated in the "comic interpretation of disaster" in the movie *Caldofreddo*, which shocks Charlie with its effectiveness. He and Humboldt argued at the time they wrote the original scenario; Humboldt maintained that "it would be extremely funny. And so it was. The plane sank. Thousands of people were laughing" (461). It "did nothing about brutality or inhumanity" and "didn't clarify much or prevent anything"; still there was "something in it" that "was pleasing hundreds of thousands, millions of spectators" (462). Charlie envisions "humanity either laughing its head off as pictures of man-eating comedy unrolled on the screen or vanishing in great waves of death, in flames and battle agonies, in starving continents" and realizes—although Humboldt eventually was overcome by the tragic aspects of his own personality—he, Charlie, is not yet ready to give up. He will "fly on" (462).

Bellow uses the character of Von Humboldt Fleisher to exemplify the theory that the weakness of comedy lies in the fact that—when the laughing stops—there still exists a big surplus of pain. Humboldt, a self-diagnosed manic-depressive, behaves like an "eccentric and a comic subject" taking an occasional break during which he stopped and thought: "He was a great entertainer but going insane. The pathological element could be missed only by those who were laughing too hard to look" (5-6). Afflicted with Pagliacci Gangrene, he complains of being "out of kilter" after having lost his equilibrium through anxiety (128).

By the time his lawyers have negotiated for an agreeable settlement with the producers of *Caldofreddo*, Charlie has finally arrived at the stage described in Point Six. After realizing that the "ideas of the last few centuries are used up" (250), Charlie gets rid of the old jokes; he rejects two very lucrative offers from the company that bought the rights to *Treatment* (482) and severs his relationship with Cantabile (483).

Charlie makes plans to join Kathleen and perhaps work as an extra in the movie *Memoirs of a Cavalier*. Confident that these "things he has to do" will be able to "find their way around those mountains of absurdities" (478), Charlie is ready to launch his new search for humanhood.

Convinced that "human beings are far too deep in that false unnecessary comedy of history," Charlie plans to look at life and his fellowman on a "different scale," a scale that would place humans on a "point within a great hierarchy that goes far beyond ourselves" (478–79). Long ago Charlie learned that "matters of the spirit are widely and instantly grasped except by those mental opponents who are trained to resist what everyone is born knowing" (91). He is now aware that mankind's escape from the "suffocation" of tragedy lies in its refusal to surrender the one element that sets man apart from the lesser animals. "The existence of a soul is beyond proof under the ruling premises, but people go on behaving as though they had souls, nevertheless" (479). As long as this behavior continues, so will man. And so will comedy.

Thus, in *Humboldt's Gift*, Bellow proves that his new New Comedy is every bit as valid and as applicable as Menander's New Comedy. However, there still remains the question of why *The Last Analysis* was not a successful stage play.

Perhaps the answer lies in the audiences. The audiences who attended and appreciated Menander's plays at the festival of Dionysus in ancient Greece knew that—dictated by tradition—Menander's plots would develop along certain lines, observe certain conventions, and be resolved in much the same fashion from play to play. In other words, they knew what to expect before they arrived at the theater. However, the audiences who attended Bellow's play did not have any such prior knowledge.

Perhaps the answer lies in the plays. Menander's plays include a prologue—usually no later than in the second scene—that tells the audience what is taking place (Murray 112). Menander's plays are, therefore, somewhat self-explanatory. Not only does *The Last Analysis* omit this element of self-explanation, it teems with Bellow's rapid dialogue, which is accompanied by quickly moving action. More than one exposure is required before an audience—theater or reading—can understand the development of the play.

Perhaps the answer lies in the playwrights themselves. Menander knew for whom he was writing as he wrote his plays. He knew his audience would expect certain elements in each play and those elements were always provided for them. Bellow did not have that advantage. An established novelist writing his first full-length stage play, Bellow took what had worked so well for years—his wit—and transferred it to the stage without alteration or explanation. Menander's genius was his ability to write playable plays for theater audiences. Bellow's genius is his ability to write readable novels for reading audiences.

Bellow's theory of comedy—developed in *The Last Analysis* and refined in *Humboldt's Gift*—updates Menander's New Comedy and restructures it to suit the tastes of the modern audience. Perhaps Bellow will go still further and actually develop the project conceived by Charlie Citrine. *The Intellectual Comedy of the Modern Mind* would not only once again confirm Bellow's theory of Sublime Comedy, it would give his readers a wonderful opportunity to once again enjoy Bellow's genius.

WORKS CITED

Bellow, Saul. *Humboldt's Gift*. New York: Viking, 1975.

---. *The Last Analysis. Comedy: A Critical Anthology*. Ed. Robert W. Corrigan. Boston: Houghton, 1971. 670–737.

Bergson, Henri. "Laughter." *Comedy: A Critical Anthology*. Ed. Robert W. Corrigan. Boston: Houghton, 1971. 745–50.

Biffle, Kent. "Mr. Bellow's Planet." *Dallas Morning News* 14 Nov. 1976: G1.

Dutton, Robert R. *Saul Bellow*. Boston: Twayne, 1971.

Holman, C. Hugh. *A Handbook to Literature*. 4th ed. Indianapolis: Bobbs, 1981. 433.

Loney, Glenn M. Headnote. *The Last Analysis*. By Saul Bellow. *Comedy: A Critical Anthology*. Ed. Robert W. Corrigan. Boston: Houghton, 1971. 670.

Malin, Irving. "Bummy's Analysis." *Saul Bellow: A Collection of Critical Essays*. Ed. Earl Rovit. Englewood Cliffs: Prentice, 1975. 115–21.

Murray, Gilbert, ed. and trans. *Two Plays of Menander:* The Rape of the Locks *and* The Arbitration. New York: Oxford UP, 1945.

Scheer-Schäzler, Brigitte. *Saul Bellow*. New York: Frederick Ungar, 1972.

Bellow's Canadian Beginnings

Michael Greenstein
University of Sherbrooke, Sherbrooke, Quebec

Augie March's author is a Canadian, Quebec born. No one overlooks the fact of Saul Bellow's Canadian birth, but what has gone unnoticed is the place of his Montreal childhood, with its multilingual environment, in his fiction. Whether the gray Arctic silence of Newfoundland is for Henderson either a point of reentry to America or an antidote to the tropical tribalism of Africa, Canada plays a role in more than one of Bellow's novels. When the Nobel Prize winner refuses the category of American Jewish writer, it is all too tempting for Canadians to want a piece of his acclaim, a portion of his birthright.

From the outset of his career with *Dangling Man*, Bellow announces: "I am still Canadian, a British subject," despite his residence in Chicago for 18 years. Just as Joseph's Jewish sensibility sets him apart through his inner-directed journal, so his Montreal roots are another source of his dangling between diverse worlds. His entry for January 5 takes the reader back to Joseph's origins, and although Bellow devotes only two paragraphs to his background, his descriptions are sufficiently detailed to prepare for developments in *Herzog* 20 years later. On this wintry afternoon Joseph empties the closet of all its shoes and sits on the floor polishing them: Bellow simultaneously empties some of his ghosts from the same closet while he polishes his prose. If *madeleines* take Proust back to his childhood, then shoes are appropriate vehicles for a dangling man searching for lost time. Chicago's rags lead to a remembrance of things past. "In Montreal, on such afternoons as this, I often asked permission to spread a paper on the sitting-room floor and shine all the shoes in the house" (57). For the child, shoe-shining is an all-encompassing activity, not just a synecdoche for human activity, but a pastime to include all members of the family. The long tongues and scores of eyelets personify Aunt Dina's shoes, while Bellow's tactile imagination penetrates to the depths of a seemingly commonplace occurrence. Up to his elbows in soft leather, with tongue in cheek and foot in mouth, Bellow tricks clichés in his supple prose.

The dialectic of dangling between interior and exterior
continues in the description of St. Dominique Street's brown fog
in contrast to the warmth of the room: outside, a slum between
market and hospital, corruption and healing; inside, a haven of
work and sensations. A fallen horse, a funeral passing through
the snow, and a cripple taunting his brother remind the reader
of urban decadence and the necessity of mending shoes for
mobility, of superimposing a cleaner surface on chaos. The
pungency of its stores and cellars, the French and immigrant
women, and the beggars with sores and deformities prepare Joseph
for his later reading about Villon's Paris. Montreal provides an
apprenticeship for Chicago's midwest frontier as well as an easterly
return to European history. "I sometimes think it is the only
place where I was ever allowed to encounter reality" (86). Amidst
this hyper-reality Joseph's father is concerned lest his son see too
much, and he does indeed witness sexual scenes from his window.
What impress the child most, however, are "a cage with a rat
in it thrown on a bonfire, and two quarreling drunkards, one
of whom walked away bleeding, drops falling from his head
like the first slow drops of a heavy rain in summer, a crooked
line of drops left on the pavement as he walked" (86). The boy
is caged in warmth and safety while the rat burns; the wounded
drunkard staggers while Joseph cleans boots and shoes, erasing
residual filth from that same pavement.

Montreal's uprooted footsteps continue to dangle on Bellow's
memory in *Herzog*. With thoughts shooting out all over the place,
trespassing on history, Herzog recalls biblical passages (about
Solomon and the lilies of the field) learned from a Christian lady
in Montreal's Royal Victoria Hospital. From his hospital bed eight-
year-old Moses spies icicles while "the goyische lady" questions
him about his background on Napoleon Street. During this
catechism Moses conceals the truth about his bootlegging father,
adhering to his mother's injunction, " 'You must never say' "
(23). Montreal and biblical instruction—whether from Old or New
Testaments, rabbis or goyische ladies—belong to Bellow's "ancient
system, of greater antiquity than the Jews themselves" (22).
Bellow's alter ego, M. E. Herzog, must somehow say the truth
about the fall from Russian "gentility" to Canadian bootlegging,
servitude, and shoe-shining.

Dodging traffic in New York and thinking about a flight in
Poland, Herzog turns his nomadic mind back 40 years to another
form of transportation:

> Anyway, a holiday should begin with a train ride, as it had when
> he was a kid in Montreal. The whole family took the streetcar to
> the Grand Trunk Station with a basket (frail, splintering wood)
> of pears, overripe, a bargain bought by Jonah Herzog at the Rachel
> Street Market, the fruit spotty, ready for wasps, just about to decay,
> but marvelously fragrant. (32)

Skidding between Grand Central and Penn Station, Herzog's
overripe mind contrasts with the decadent still life even as his
father's Russian knife and European efficiency clash with the worn
seats, soot, and grimy weeds. Crossing the St. Lawrence or any
other river of the Diaspora with his acute memories, Moses drives
his cart and plow over the bones of the dead from Russia back to
the Bible. His mother's handkerchief wiping his face clean of soot
and pear juice cannot erase the memory of the Canadian station.
Through the narrow perspective of window or toilet funnel, the
child observes the frothing river, the Lachine Rapids, and the
Indian reservation at Caughnawaga. Bellow's Canadian landscape
serves as a rite of passage or training ground for his entry into
an adult's America.

Surveying New York from "the middle height" and human
nature from a higher loft, Herzog writes a letter to his old friend
from Montreal's slums—Nachman of Napoleon Street. Herzog
had recently spotted his friend of 40 years running away from
him on 8th St.; this flight of Nachman the poet is characteristic
once again of Herzog's own fugitive mind, building Versailles
as well as Jerusalem in Ludeyville. Gone are Aristotelian unities
and in their place Bellow substitutes 40 years of cerebral wan-
dering across frozen deserts and promised lands. Between Montreal
and New York, Moses recalls an incident in Paris when Nachman
had borrowed money from him to return to America. These
incidents in turn spark earlier memories of their childhood in
North America's Parisian equivalent: "But we did play in the
street together. I learned the *aleph-beth* from your father, Reb
Shika" (131). Herzog's ironic Hasidism derives from Rabbi
Nachman of Bratslav even as his gutter alphabet prepares him
for exile in Chicago. Five-year-old Moses crosses Napoleon Street
and eventually the borders of cosmopolitanism, chased not so
much by Pharoah's chariots as by memories of fallen peddlers'
horses and *yichus* (a Yiddish system of reward and achievement).
Instead of Sinai, he climbs up a "wooden staircase with slanted,
warped treads. Cats shrank into corners or bolted softly upstairs.
Their dry turds crumbled in the darkness with a spicy odor."

Centuries of ghetto life cling to Bellow's naturalism, Montreal's tenement contrasting with New York's highrise, for we are never in one place or one time in multilayered *Herzog*. "Reb Shika had a yellow color, Mongolian, a tiny handsome man. He wore a black satin skullcap, a mustache like Lenin's. . . . The Bible lay open on the coarse table cover. Moses clearly saw the Hebrew characters—DMAI OCHICHO—the blood of thy brother. Yes, that was it. God speaking to Cain" (131). In ironic juxtapositions of cat and Shika, Lenin and Bible, New World and Old Testament, Nachman's blood and tears cry out to Bellow who clearly sees his Hebrew characters.

In the cellar of the synagogue Moses and Nachman share a bench and lessons from a rabbi who translates from the original Hebrew and predicts that his lazy pupils will grow up to eat pork. Future poet and historian take refuge in the primitive W.C. where disinfectant camphor balls dwindle in the green trough of the urinal, and old purblind men from the shul grumble liturgy as they wait for redemptive waters. As a way station between the old and the new, Europe and the U.S., the Bible and the modern novel, cellars and upward mobility, Canada is a good training ground for aspiring Jewish poets and historians of Romanticism. Side by side with two Nachmans are two Herzogs and at least as many Bellows with their cold pastorals.

Nachman writes his New Psalms and reminds Moses of the old poverty of Uncle Ravitch, the drunkard, who worked at the fruit store near Rachel Street in 1922. A melancholy loner trying to send for his family in Russia, Ravitch drinks his pay and judges himself harshly, so the Herzogs pity him and take him in as a boarder. Sharing a bed with his brothers Willie and Shura, Moses observes the nocturnal scene of his father helping Ravitch, who resembles a tragic actor on the Yiddish stage, while Father Herzog in his Russian linen sleeping suit recalls a "gentlemanly" Petersburg past. This closet drama of Ravitch wailing his Hebrew and Yiddish lines is played against a domestic backdrop of the empty kitchen. "The black cookstove against the wall, extinct; the double gas ring connected by rubber pipe to the meter. A Japanese reed mat protected the wall from cooking stains" (136). A stopover between Petersburg and Chicago, Montreal's Jewish kitchen is all but extinct, part of the changed condition between Russia and America.

This picture of pathetic Ravitch chanting " '*Al tastir ponecho mimeni*' " (Do not hide Thy countenance from us) leads to a portrait of Jonah Herzog as Bellow plays God in revealing various countenances. Whether stropping his bone-handled razors, sharpening pencils on the ball of his thumb, holding a loaf of bread to his breast and slicing toward himself, or jotting like an artist in his account book, Jonah performs dexterously with Eastern European flourishes in the old system's slice of life. But his artistic gestures end in failure, first in Russia, then in Canada, swallowed by continental leviathans. In 1913 he fails as a farmer in Valleyfield, Quebec, to be followed by successive failures as baker, jobber, junk dealer, marriage broker, and bootlegger. Montreal's middleman rushes around, his coat "sweeping open as he walked, or marched his one-man Jewish march, he was saturated with the odor of the Caporals he smoked as he covered Montreal in his swing—Papineau, Mile-End, Verdun, Lachine, Point St. Charles" (137). To Petersburg, Napoleon Street, and a biblical Rachel Street, Augie March's ancestor adds new territories outside ghetto regionalism. Moses inherits his father's nomadism but turns it inward, replacing space with the one-man procession in history and old poverty.

Tracing his Loman lineage even further, he turns next to Grandfather Herzog, who took refuge in the Winter Palace in 1918. With his instinct for "the grand thing" and his long letters in elegant Hebrew calligraphy, he transmits a "high style" to his son and a metaphysics to his grandson. The vast ocean that separates generations of Herzogs contrasts with Montreal's cave-like kitchen, its ancient black stove the center of Moses' world. (Even in Ludeyville, the kitchen becomes his headquarters for writing his random thoughts.) From the primitive kitchen the narrator turns naturally to a portrait of Mother Herzog, who meets the present with a partly averted face, partly because reality is too hard to bear, partly in response to the "concealed countenance" in " '*Al tastir ponecho mimeni.*' " On her withdrawn side "she often had a dreaming look, melancholy, and seemed to be seeing the Old World—her father the famous *misnagid*, her tragic mother . . . and her linens and servants in Petersburg, the dacha in Finland (all founded on Egyptian onions)" (139). Napoleon Street represents a mighty falling for this New World cook, washerwoman, and seamstress who has lost so much. Moses inherits this loss, equal portions of the romantic *hasid* and rational *misnagid*, Mediterranean bulrushes and onions; his early training in ancient and medieval history serves him well in his later studies of the seventeenth and eighteenth centuries in *Romanticism and Christianity*. Montreal's averted neo-Victorian aspect connects earlier centuries to the twentieth and turns back the clock.

Its frozen withdrawn side exists at the opposite pole of the world from those ill-founded Egyptian onions. "My ancient times. Remoter than Egypt. No dawn, the foggy winters." A pervasive darkness covers snow and daylight, and in the midst of gloom, dung, and dead rats Moses prays: " 'How goodly are thy tents, O Israel.' " This yawning gap between Zion's prayers and Montreal's reality invites Bellow's irony, the age-old disjunction between chosenness and persecution, and leads immediately to the apostrophe, "Napoleon Street, rotten, toylike, crazy and filthy, riddled, flogged with harsh weather—the bootlegger's boys reciting ancient prayers" (140). With only one direction to go in, brother Shura will master the world to become a millionaire, sister Helen at the piano will play Haydn and Mozart *avec distinction*, and Herzog himself (under a slightly different guise) will bring the Nobel Prize home to Napoleon Street.

> To this Moses' heart was attached with great power. Here was a wider range of human feelings than he had ever again been able to find. The children of the race, by a never-failing miracle, opened their eyes on one strange world after another, age after age, and uttered the same prayer in each, eagerly loving what they found. What was wrong with Naopleon Street? thought Herzog. All he ever wanted was there. (140)

The paradox of Herzog's heartache centers on Napoleon Street or St. Dominique: the narrower the ghetto, the wider the emotions; the more particular or parochial Montreal's slum, the more universal its significance. Helen's music and Bellow's cadences ring into the street, transcending the trails of ashes with "heart-rotting emotions, black spots, sweet for one moment but leaving a dangerous acid residue" (141). Lost and found diasporic shifts from Petersburg to Montreal to Chicago make ambivalence inevitable.

Now a British subject beyond the Pale, Uncle Yaffe wears a beard like King George V (the Czar's cousin) and labors at the Canadian Pacific Railways before owning a junkyard in St. Anne where Indians from Caughnawaga come to trade. His wife, Aunt Zipporah, collects rents, becomes rich, and accuses Moses' parents of behaving as if they still belonged to a higher class in Russia. Her junkyard wealth contrasts with her family's silk-shirted, *edel* poverty, values of old and new worlds. " 'I can still see you getting off the train from Halifax, all dressed up among the greeners.

Gott meiner! Ostrich feathers, taffeta skirts! *Greenhorns mit strauss federn*!' " (142). Since Zipporah's name means "bird," the irony of those feathers is directed back at her, even as her branch of the family will join the vulgar ranks of the nouveau riche while Jonah's offspring, descending from Hasidic rabbis, know a page of *Gemara* or the notes of Mozart. What differentiates their arrival in Halifax from immigration to Ellis Island is a slower process of assimilation within the Canadian mosaic rather than the American melting pot. If, as Moses thinks, one of life's hardest jobs is to make a quick understanding slow, then the Canadian experience retards the immigrant's entry before the rush to New York or Chicago. Where Emma Lazarus' words welcomed huddled masses at Ellis Island before thrusting them into American culture already established in the nineteenth century, no strong indigenous culture was in place to the north so that Bellow's family clung to its Yiddish roots somewhat longer than if it had arrived directly south of the border. Those few formative years in Montreal with its French Catholic and Anglo-Presbyterian solitudes made a difference, translating French and Yiddish.

Bellow haunts the past on a winter day in 1923 in Aunt Zipporah's St. Anne kitchen. During their Yiddish conversation, the Herzogs always refer to Russia as *in der heim*—a homeless home where Jonah at least did not have to shovel manure. Escaping from the Czar's police he now evades the Revenue with his still in the land of Columbus. The little Canadian village can barely contain an ambitious Zipporah with her large hips, bosom stuffed with a bankroll, and opinionated voice. Whenever the children are sick, Aunt Zipporah brings an egg wrapped in Yiddish newspaper (*Der Kanader Adler*), for she is a hard-boiled realist unlike Herzog's mystical mother. The humiliation of Shura pasting labels on bottles of bootleg whiskey and the sight of Jonah beaten up on the way to the border bears an uncanny resemblance to Dickens' experiences at the blacking factory. No borders would stand in the way of Jonah's son and creator on the road to international recognition. The Baron de Hirsch school forms part of Herzog's *Bildung*, but his schooling in grief goes back further to "Jewish antiquities originating in the Bible, in a Biblical sense of personal experience and destiny" (148).

Exaggerating slightly, Leon Edel has written:

> In the streets of Montreal, on cold winter days, you could meet, in the 1920's, characters wrapped in great coats, their breath exhaled in vapor, walking out of the 19th century—in Westmount out of

> Dickens or Thackeray, in Montreal East out of Balzac. And in
> between, figures Biblical, or characters created by say Israel
> Zangwill—a glimpse of the Galician or Rumanian, the Lithuanian,
> or the Russian. (17–18)

Although Edel is referring to the work of A. M. Klein, his words
apply equally to Bellow, who carries this tradition further into
the twentieth century. In *The Second Scroll* and in his poem
"Autobiographical," Klein draws on many of the same Montreal
images as Bellow. Bellow's brief residence in Montreal places
him not only with Klein but with Mordecai Richler and Leonard
Cohen, who have devoted their careers to St. Urbain's setting.
"I am a Canadian, too, you know," writes Herzog in one of his
final letters (315). Bellow is a citizen of the world, an American,
Canada-born, a particular universalist and denizen of the Diaspora
whose stay in Montreal made a difference *avec distinction* and
yichus. In Canadian cellars and junkyards Bellow doffed his
Russian finery before outfitting himself at Hart, Schaffner, and
Marx; unshod for a time, with his foot in his mouth, he tested
the cold waters of the St. Lawrence before entering the American
mainstream. Augie March was not the first to knock because Mark
Twain had already scouted the Mississippi; on the St. Lawrence,
Moses Herzog's only precursors were non-Canadian Hebrew,
Yiddish, and French patriarchs who followed him across the Great
Lakes. Only in North America could a Chicago Yankee knock
at King George's and King Solomon's courts.

WORKS CITED

Bellow, Saul. *Dangling Man*. New York: Avon, 1980.
———. *Herzog*. New York: Viking, 1964.
Edel, Leon. "Marginal *Keri* and Textual *Chetiv*: The Mythic Novel of
    A. M. Klein." In *The A. M. Klein Symposium*. Ed. Seymour Mayne.
    Ottawa: U of Ottawa P, 1975.

Saul Bellow:
Sojourner in New York

David D. Anderson
Michigan State University

Saul Bellow's novel, *Dangling Man*, is a city novel but not a novel of the city, a novel set in Chicago but not of Chicago; it is a war novel but not a novel about the war; it is a novel about apparent choices when in reality there are none; it is a novel about a young man who seeks isolation but ultimately accepts absorption into "the uniform of the times," knowing that a separate peace is impossible, that his concern must be with what he calls *le genre humain*, that he will ultimately accept the fact of his victimization as he accepts the fact of war and the responsibility of his generation.

At this point Bellow begins his second novel, *The Victim*. Like its predecessor, it is a city novel—Bellow's first set in New York—but it is not a New York novel; it is a post-war, post-holocaust novel that is about neither; it is a novel about a man approaching middle age who seeks to escape victimization and duty and responsibility, all of which he sees as synonymous, but he finds they are not. But while *Dangling Man* ends on a note of reluctant acceptance of an inevitable dehumanization, *The Victim* affirms a common humanity.

Bellow begins *The Victim* with a technical device that he had not used in *Dangling Man* and was not to use again in a novel. It is used here, I suspect, because the ending of *Dangling Man* continues to test critical arts and insights, and Bellow wanted no such problem in *The Victim*. But the device—two epigraphs—makes the price of literary clarity too high as it gives away too much at the beginning.

The first epigraph, from *The Thousand and One Nights*, tells of a merchant who pauses on his journey to rest and eat, throwing away his date pits with force. Suddenly a huge Ifrit appears, brandishing a sword, and tells the merchant, " 'Stand up that I may slay thee even as thou slewest my son!' " The merchant, confused, asks, " 'How have I slain thy son?' " and the Ifrit replies, " 'When thou atest dates and threwest away the stones

they struck my son full in the breast as he was walking by, so
that he died forthwith.' "

The second epigraph, from DeQuincey's *The Pains of Opium*,
is an image of the surging ocean as it turns into a human face
and then "innumerable faces, upturned to the heavens; faces,
imploring, wrathful, despairing; faces that surged upward by
thousands, by myriads, by generations. . . ."

The first epigraph suggests the complexity of the extent of
human responsibility for human actions and the ambiguity of
the line between guilt and innocence; the second, the complexity
of the relationship between the individual and the mass and the
inevitability of human suffering.

The epigraphs combine to suggest the position of Asa
Leventhal, the novel's protagonist, as the novel opens. Asa, like
Joseph of *Dangling Man*, is alone in the mass of Manhattan rather
than the Southside neighborhood of Chicago. Like Joseph, he
is dangling at loose ends while his wife Mary visits her mother
in the South. A largely self-taught editor, he works on a trade
publication. He has a few acquaintances, fewer friends, a brother's
family in distress on Staten Island, and chronic job insecurity.
Unlike Joseph, who is ethnically uncertain but vaguely Christian,
Asa is clearly ethnically a non-practicing Jew.

The opening chapter defines the three dimensions of Asa's
predicament: "New York is as hot as Bangkok" (3) as Asa returns
from his sister-in-law's flat on Staten Island. He had been called
there by his hysterical Italian sister-in-law, Elena. His brother Max
is working in Galveston; their baby is ill; can he come? He does,
although the journal is about to go to press, and he is needed
in the office. As he leaves, he overhears an anti-Semitic tirade
from his boss. By the time he gets there, the baby is better, and
he returns home in the heat, narrowly escaping being caught in
the door of a Third Avenue train. Asa, cursing as he descends
the stairs, is not only the victimized modern man in the city, the
individual in an oppressive naturalistic environment, and the Jew
in the gentile world; he is, as his name makes clear, Asa, the
dutiful if reluctant healer.

Asa has known good times and bad. He had enjoyed an
idyllic time in Baltimore as a customs agent, where he met Mary,
and after a quarrel returned to New York. There, in the midst
of a depression, he luckily found work. After two years, he and
Mary were married. Occasionally, remembering his good fortune,
he told her, " 'I was lucky. I got away with it' " (20)

Circumstances, in other words, might easily have destroyed him, but somehow they had worked out in his favor. Yet he is not a happy man; his days and nights are full of guilt, responsibility, and resentment, all intensified during Mary's absence.

From this point Bellow develops two plot lines. The first, apparently the lesser, defines Asa's relationship with his brother's family and the combination of duty, resentment, and guilt with which he tries to bring order to a chaotic situation, build a dutiful bridge to an older nephew, see that the baby has medical care, allay Elena's and Elena's mother's real or imagined resentment toward him as a Jew and an outsider, force Max's return to his family, and imbue him with suitable measures of responsibility and guilt.

The second plot line develops Leventhal's relationship with Kirby Allbee, a former acquaintance who comes out of his past, accusing, blaming, and, like the Ifrit, threatening. Allbee insists that Asa had caused him to lose his editorial job, thereby triggering a series of personal disasters—his wife's leaving him, her death in a traffic accident, dissipation with the insurance money, and now destitution. Allbee insists he is Asa's victim, and he demands an unnamed reparation, his accusations laced with genteel but no less offensive anti-Semitism.

As Allbee haunts Asa on the streets and in his flat, moves in with him, and finally subjects him to the ultimate indignity of bringing a whore to Asa and Mary's bed, perhaps hoping that Asa would return and find them (Asa does and is torn between resentment and a desire to laugh at a naked, overweight Allbee handing stockings to a naked, overweight whore), Asa insists that he is not guilty. Then he isn't sure. Ultimately he concedes to himself that he may be guilty or partially guilty, and begins to inquire about possible jobs for Allbee.

The beginning of Allbee's downfall and the source of Asa's guilt was an incident that occurred shortly after Asa's return from Baltimore. They met at a party given by mutual acquaintances, and Allbee agreed to arrange an interview with his employer, Rudiger, owner of a journal called *Dill's Weekly*. In the interview, Asa found Rudiger offensive; tired, frustrated, and angry, Asa was abusive in return. The memory of the incident had, over the years, bothered him from time to time. Allbee tells Asa that he was fired shortly after that incident and that the connection is clear: Asa had unleashed the firing in a series of connected incidents; Asa was responsible and guilty.

As Asa moved through what had become a circumscribed routine—sleep filled with threatening dreams, solitary meals in a nearby Italian restaurant, the strains of work, journeys to Staten Island, jousts with the masses (Asa's most frequent human encounters), and his sessions with Allbee—the two plots move toward their climaxes and resolutions. The brother's baby, suddenly worse, is hospitalized at Asa's insistence and against Elena's judgment and treated by a doctor secured by Asa. The baby goes into a coma and then dies. Max arrives typically too late.

Asa cries when he hears the news; he fears that Elena will blame him for the disease, the hospital, the doctor, the death. He exchanges meaningless words with Max, silently endures a Catholic burial service, and then finds himself alone in the crowded park near his flat:

> The trees were swathed in stifling dust, and the stars were faint and sparse through the pall. The benches formed a dense double human wheel; the paths were thronged. There was an overwhelming human closeness and thickness, and Leventhal was penetrated by a sense not merely of the crowd in the park but of innumerable millions, crossing, toughing, pressing. What was that story he had once read about Hell cracking open on account of the rage of the sea, and all the souls, crammed together, looking out? But these were alive, this young couple with bare arms, this woman late in pregnancy, sauntering, this bootblack hauling his box by the long strap. (183–84)

Asa remembers the day, thinks of his father, who would find it incomprehensible, and then, exhausted, returns to the flat. Allbee's earlier departure, in flight, following his whore, is for Asa the end of a nightmare, and yet Asa wonders as he looks about the flat:

> "Maybe I didn't do the right thing. I didn't know what it was. I don't yet. And there had to be a showdown sooner or later. What was I going to do with him? He hated me. He hated me enough to cut my throat. He didn't do it because he was too much of a coward. . . . He hated himself for not having enough nerve. . . . I had to do somethng with him. I suppose I handled it badly." (277)

As he begins to straighten up after the mess of Allbee's visit, Leventhal's thoughts echo his earlier revelations to Mary: " 'Still, it's over,' " he tells himself; " 'that's the main thing.' " He opens a can of soup and turns on the radio for the company of another voice. The phone rings; it's his brother to tell him he is on his way over.

Max's visit is short and unstrained. He has convinced Elena to return to Galveston with him; he has just picked up reservations at Penn Station; they will leave on Friday; Asa promises to see them off. Then he calls Mary. She will leave the next day and be home in the morning.

As Asa sleeps, he dreams of the odor and color of cosmetics; half-awake, he remembers the whore in his bed, and is suddenly awake, recognizing the smell of gas. In the kitchen he grasps the figure he knows is Allbee; they struggle, and Allbee flees into the night. Asa, shaken, turns off the gas and opens the windows. Was Allbee committing suicide, as he insisted he was? Or murder and suicide? Or simply murder? Asa barricades the door, notices the chair in front of the stove, and goes back to bed, to sleep dreamlessly but well. Allbee is gone from his life, Mary will return in a day, Max's family is together, and he can pick up the strands of his life.

Mary returns, fall comes, time passes, a better job comes, Asa begins to gray, Mary becomes pregnant, all in the coda that is the last chapter. Asa loses his sense of guilty relief, of having gotten away with it, and he recognizes the haphazard quality of life, the accidental nature of success and failure that denies either justice or injustice. He comes to believe, too, that there are more important dimensions of life to be found, "more important things to be promised" (286), although he hasn't yet achieved them, indeed does not yet understand them. On occasion he wonders what happened to Allbee and he hears vague rumors, all of them different: Allbee is institutionalized, hospitalized, dead in some Potter's Field. He chooses not "to think too much or too literally about it" (287). He has made his peace with himself.

One scene remains: on a hot June evening Asa and Mary go to a Broadway play. As they enter the theater, Mary recognizes a fading actress; Asa recognizes the actress's companion, an older, more presentable Allbee in a dinner jacket. During the intermission they meet; the conversation is strained:

> "I want you to know one thing," said Allbee. "That night . . . I wanted to put an end to myself. I wasn't thinking of hurting you. . . . You weren't even in my mind."
> Leventhal laughed outright at this.
> "You could have jumped in the river. That's a funny lie. Why tell it? Did you have to use my kitchen?"
> "No," he said miserably. . . . "I must have been demented. . . . But I want to say I owe you something. . . . I know I owe you. . . ." (293)

Mutually embarrassed, they change topics. Allbee is in radio advertising, a minor functionary. " 'I'm not the type who runs things,' " he says. " 'What do I care? The world wasn't made exactly for me.' "

Allbee turns back to the theater, and Asa cries out, " 'Wait a minute, what's your idea of who runs things?' " (294). But he hears Mary's voice, they return to their seats in the dark as the lights go out, and the novel ends on an unanswered, unanswerable question.

Allbee and Asa have each made their peace with life and circumstance, and they have made peace with each other. In the scene they might have been old friends, and yet the final question remains, answerable not only in the hot, oppressive naturalistic atmosphere of both beginning and end, but in the epigraphs of the faces, not individual but one, and of the Ifrit who proclaims guilt when there is instead a mutual responsibility.

Much critical attention has been devoted to three aspects of the novel: the real, imagined, and feared anti-Semitism, which some see as the central theme of the novel; the overt Dreiserian naturalism of the city as setting and force; and the influence of Dostoyevski, especially his novellas *The Eternal Husband* and *The Double* on the novel's structure and plot. Some critics have insisted that it is Bellow's most Jewish novel, pointing for evidence not only to the frequent usages, idioms, and rhythms that echo the Yiddish, but also to the angst and affirmation that alternate and then become one.

Bellow himself has acknowledged the debt to Dostoyevski, although insisting he was unaware of it when he wrote. But he has also pointed out, "I was doing nothing very original by writing another realistic novel about a common man and calling it *The Victim*" ("Saul Bellow" 61). But both the general critical comments and Bellow's self-effacing remarks overlook the subtlety and complexity of Bellow's first major excursion into modernism.

Each of the critical generalizations has in it part of the truth. Anti-Semitism, real or imagined, is central to Asa's relationships with Allbee, with Elena, with his boss Mr. Beard, even with the nameless hordes on the streets and the mechanical monsters that permit the city to function. Those same relationships also give focus to Asa's self-image as victim. But Bellow makes it clear that although Asa has experienced anti-Semitic abuse, it is the abuse of the nightmare that is the city, and he has never known overt discrimination. Furthermore, just as Asa sees himself as Allbee's victim, Allbee sees himself as the victim of the circumstances set into motion by Asa's unpleasant act and hence Asa's victim, further victimized through the loss of WASP power and prestige in a changing society. Allbee emphasizes that he, a descendent of Governor Winthrop, has been vicitmized by what he calls a Jewish "set-up," just as Asa has feared the invoking of an anti-Jewish blacklist against him. But there is neither "set-up" nor blacklist, although neither can see the truth. While Asa sees himself as a Jew and a victim, and Allbee sees himself as a gentile, equally a victim, it is evident that each is a victim only in his own mind and in the human nature they share.

Real victims do exist in the novel, but neither man knows or sees them except in the mass. Early in the novel Asa finds himself grateful that he never became one of "the lost, the outcast, the overcome, the effaced, the ruined" who sleep under bridges or on park benches. But he doesn't see the city's victims when they approach him. In one instance, as he lunches with acquaintances, "a Filipino busboy came to clear the table. He was an old man and frail looking, and his hands and forearms were whitened by immersions in hot water. The cart loaded, he bent his back low over it, receiving the handlebar in his chest, and pushed away slowly . . . " (130). But Asa, engaged in a discussion of Disraeli as Jew, doesn't notice him.

The source of each man's sense of victimization lies in his inability to see the moral ties of a mutual responsibility that bind each to the other. Consequently, Asa is torn between guilt and duty—guilt in his treatment of Allbee, duty toward his brother's family—and an inability or refusal to accept responsibility willingly for either. And Allbee proclaims his own denial of responsibility:

> "We don't choose much. We don't choose to be born, for example, and unless we commit suicide we don't choose the time to die, either. . . . The world's a crowded place, damned if it isn't. . . . Do you want anything? . . . There are a hundred million others who want that same thing. I don't care whether it's a sandwich or a seat in the subway or what. . . . Who wants all these people to be here . . . ?" (193–94)

There is clearly much of Dostoyevski here, especially of the psychic pairing of *The Double.* But Bellow takes it beyond Dostoyevski and into a redoubled, even a tripled, psychic mirroring as each—Asa, Allbee, Max—learns from the other about the ties that bind them, the ties of a common humanity as well as ties of blood. At one point, Asa cries out to Allbee, " 'What,

are we related?' '' And Allbee laughs, '' 'By blood? No, no' ''
(29). Yet it becomes clear that they are.

Ultimately the pattern of moral judgment, of projecting guilt
on others, gives way to an acceptance of responsibility. This guilt
is purged; hatred, real and imagined, is dissipated; and perceptions that had threatened to become stereotypes, the goy seen
by Asa and the yid seen by Allbee, disappear. Simultaneously,
new mutual perceptions emerge. Final encounters, of Asa and
Max, of Asa and Allbee, suggest that each, in accepting responsibility not only for others but for himself, accepts his share of
a common humanity, a common responsibility, and emerges with
a kind of dignity he had not known before.

It is this sense of dignity, of intrinsic human worth, that
Bellow suggests is the only knowable end of human life. Asa's
lunch with friends includes the speech of an otherwise extraneous
character in a nearly extraneous incident. While the Filipino
busboy goes through his chores in unnoticed and unstudied
dignity, Mr. Schlossberg, a writer who writes ''everything'' for
the Jewish press, in the longest speech in the book and one of
the longest Bellow has written, insists, in a wide-ranging conversation, that '' 'I try to give everybody credit. . . . I am not a
knocker. I am not too good for this world' ''; and again, '' 'It's
bad to be less than human and it's bad to be more than human.
. . . More than human, can you have any use for life? Less than
human, you don't either' ''; and yet again, '' 'You say less than
human, more than human. Tell me, please what is human?' ''
(133–34).

Finally, Schlossberg becomes impassioned,

> ''But I say, 'What do you know? No, tell me, what do you know?
> You shut one eye and look at a thing, and it is one way to you.
> You shut the other one and it is different. I am as sure about
> greatness and beauty as you are about black and white. If a human
> life is a great thing to me, it *is* a great thing. Do you know better?
> I'm entitled as much as you. And why be measly? Do you have
> to be? Is somebody holding you by the neck? Have dignity, you
> understand me? Choose dignity. . . .' '' (134)

The speech and the lunch end in a joke that even Schlossberg
shares, but Asa is disturbed, yet he doesn't know why. But the
speech marks the vague beginning of his freedom from his own
self-perception as a victim.

In the last scene of the novel, neither Asa nor Allbee is
completely healed. Each disappears into the dark, hot theater

interior, the ultimate, unanswerable metaphysical question still hanging in the air between them. But clearly, importantly, it doesn't matter as Bellow moves beyond philosophical inquiry to end, not in acceptance of the common uniform of appearance, but in an almost un-Jewish image that owes much to Walt Whitman and the early Sherwood Anderson, a note of traditional American optimism that was to mark much of his next novel, *The Adventures of Augie March.* Asa—and Allbee—have clearly been reborn; each is a new man risen out of the ashes of hate.

WORK CITED

Bellow, Saul. Interview. "The Art of Fiction." *Paris Review* 36: 61.

Bellow the Allegory King: Animal Imagery in *Henderson the Rain King*

Kathleen King
Idaho State University

Writers sometimes structure allegories around a quest because the reader has the reward of knowing the story on many levels. The travels of the protagonist parallel both the search for meaning in the underlying source tale and the reader's own search for meaning in life. *Henderson the Rain King* is one such novel, delightful in part because Saul Bellow covers the biblical exploits of St. John, Daniel, and Nebuchadnezzar with a clever layer of modern-day adventure.

Henderson's adventurous quest corresponds with his need to resolve his neurosis. French psychoanalyst Lacan postulates that neurosis is not knowing one's desire. Henderson's neurosis takes the form of restlessness, suffering, and the inner voice which cries "I want." When Henderson travels to Africa, faces the prophecy of Nebuchadnezzar's dream, and discovers his animal nature, he stops *becoming*, starts *being*, and finally learns what he wants.

The biblical prophecy which forms the framework of the book appears five times. At first the prophecy appears to be just another of Bellow's literary allusions. "Anyway, I was a pig man. And as the prophet Daniel warned King Nebuchadnezzar, 'They shall drive thee from among men, and thy dwelling shall be with the beasts of the field' " (21). The actual quotation to which Bellow refers appears in verse 25, chapter 4 of the Book of Daniel as Daniel interprets the dream of King Nebuchadnezzar:

> That they shall drive thee from men, and thy dwelling shall
> be with the beasts of the field, and they shall make thee to eat
> grass as oxen, and they shall wet thee with the dew of heaven,
> and seven times shall pass over thee, till thou know that the most
> High ruleth in the kingdom of men, and giveth it to whomsoever
> he will.

Unfortunately, King Nebuchadnezzar refuses to believe the interpretation, even though he asked Daniel for advice. After a voice from heaven repeats the prophecy, Nebuchadnezzar still is not convinced; however, the prophecy comes true: "The same hour was the thing fulfilled upon Nebuchadnezzar: and he was driven from men, and did eat grass as oxen, and his body was wet with the dew of heaven, till his hairs were grown like eagles' feathers, and his nails like birds' claws" (Dan. 4.33). The fulfillment of the prophecy causes Nebuchadnezzar to accept the supremacy of God and bow to His will; eventually, the king is restored to both his reason and his kingdom.

The second reference to the prophecy occurs the day before the frog massacre. The Arnewi people must have "no ahnimal in drink wattah," and because frogs have invaded their cistern, the cattle are dying of thirst (51). Seeing the frogs as the cause of the death of the Arnewi cattle, and perhaps the people as well, Henderson realizes the frogs are "fundamentally harmless little semi-fishes" (89). He admits, "I was once more fatally embroiled with animals, according to the prophecy of Daniel which I had never been able to shake off—'They shall drive you from among men, and thy dwelling shall be with the beasts of the field' " (89). Weighing the benefits and drawbacks, Henderson decides that frog souls do not equal the souls of the cattle and humans who might perish if the frogs continue to pollute the cistern.

On the night before the frog massacre, ponderous issues coil around and around in Henderson's mind, causing him to lie awake and think even harder. The prophecy surfaces a third time:

> I don't often suffer from insomnia but tonight I had a lot of things on my mind, the prophecy of Daniel, the cat, the frogs, the ancient-looking place, the weeping delegation, the wrestling match with Itelo, and the queen having looked into my heart and telling me of the grun-tu-molani. (94)

Despite his concerned thoughts, Henderson's solution backfires; his homemade bomb blows up frogs *and* cistern, destroying the Arnewi water supply, so he must leave. Once again he drives himself "from among men" out into the African wilderness.

When King Dahfu of the Wariri takes Henderson to visit Atti, the sorceress–lioness, the prophecy appears again. Henderson hears the powerful roar of the lioness and sees her sleek, muscular body, and he feels frightened and confused by the king's warm relationship with such a fierce creature:

> Once again I brought to mind that old prophecy Daniel made to Nebuchadnezzar. *They shall drive thee from among men, and*

thy dwelling shall be with the beasts of the field. The lion odor
was still very keen on my fingers. I smelled it repeatedly and there
returned to my thoughts the frogs of the Arnewi, the cattle whom
they venerated, the tenants' cat I had tried to murder, to say
nothing of the pigs I had bred. Sure enough, this prophecy had
a peculiar relevance to me, implying perhaps that I was not entirely
fit for human companionship. (229–30)

Here the prophecy helps Henderson understand that the truth
he has been searching for, the particular wisdom to answer the
voice which has so many times cried "I want, I want" can be
learned from "the beasts of the field."

Bellow draws in the prophecy a final time as Henderson takes
Dahfu's lessons in lion-ness with outward good grace and inward
disgruntlement at the picture he makes: a very large, overweight,
middle-aged man wearing dirty, sagging underwear beneath trans-
parent green trousers, down on all fours in the cage of a lioness,
roaring. If animals are the source of truth, then Henderson must
become as animal as possible. The lioness Atti, noble and loving,
is a fitting teacher. Most wonderfully, the prophecy comes true:

> And so I was the beast. I gave myself to it, and all my sorrow came
> out in the roaring. My lungs supplied the air but the note came
> from my soul. The roaring scalded my throat and hurt the corners
> of my mouth and presently I filled the den like a bass organ pipe.
> This was where my heart had sent me, with its clamor. This is where
> I ended up. Oh, Nebuchadnezzar! How well I understand that
> prophecy of Daniel. For I had claws, and hair, and some teeth,
> and I was bursting with hot noise, but when all this had come
> forth, there was still a remainder. That last thing of all was my
> human longing. (267)

Henderson realizes the one thing which separates him forever from
animals is this "human longing," the voice which cries "I want."

Creatures used in *Henderson* to illustrate the fulfillment of
the prophecy can be divided into four groups: insects; fish,
amphibians, and reptiles; birds; and mammals. Each group plays
several roles within the novel.

The locusts mentioned throughout the book are usually connected with purification. Henderson prepares himself for purification by divesting himself of worldly goods: " 'Let me throw away
my gun and my helmet and the lighter and all this stuff and
maybe I can get rid of my fierceness too and live out there on
worms. On locusts. Until all the bad is burned out of me' " (49).
When leaving the Arnewi, Henderson tries to send the faithful
Romilayu off with all his possessions, even the gun which might

insure a steady supply of food. " 'I can eat locusts,' " Henderson says. Once again he searches for purification after the frog-bombing disaster. The third mention of locusts occurs as King Dahfu and a woman who looks "like a giant locust" leap and play catch with skulls during the Wariri rainmaking ceremony (175). By the end of Henderson's African adventure, Romilayu has proven to be a valuable companion, able to find both water and food in the wilderness. The two escapees live "on locusts, like Saint John" (326). Mark 1.6 tells of John's life in the wilderness: "And John was clothed with camel's hair, and with a girdle of a skin about his loins; and he did eat locusts and wild honey." Like John, Henderson is a "voice of one crying in the wilderness" (Mark 1.3).

Spiders creep into the story with two connotations. The hair of Queen Willatale, and also that of an old native musician, is described as "a million spider lines" and "white weblike hairs" (84, 254). In both instances weblike hair correlates with great age and the personal power called grun-tu-molani, the desire to live. Henderson and Romilayu see giant spiders as they walk through the wilderness from the lands of the Arnewi to the Wariri territory (114). Later when Henderson gazes with amazement at Dahfu as the latter states his theory that " 'the noble will have its turn in the world,' " the big man describes his mood as that of a spider transformed, suddenly able "to do a treatise on botany" (215). Air currents lift spider webs hanging from the walls of the tunnel as Henderson descends to the lioness's den for the first time.

Flies are first mentioned in relation to cattle, specifically the Arnewi cattle on the day of frog doom. Twice flies buzz about an incident and Henderson's memory of it: "That's like a poem I once read called, 'Written in Prison.' I can't remember it all, but part of it goes, 'I envy e'en the fly its gleams of joy, in the green woods' and it ends, 'The fly I envy settling in the sun On the green leaf and wish my goal was won' " (190). Henderson's search for understanding of the bothersome *I want* leads him to talk in metaphors of inner peace. Later Dahfu chides Henderson gently with the fly poem when the big man appears to lose his grip on his ideals (265). Henderson also notices flies sitting on the goddess Mummah during the Wariri rainmaking ceremony (192). The flies on the Arnewi cattle and the flies on Mummah are both associated with incidents in which Henderson looses water on the world.

Less frequently mentioned insects include ants, cicadas, grubs, worms, and larvae, the basis of Henderson's starvation diet during his John-like wilderness experience. Perhaps the most interesting insect is the maggot which crawls out of the decaying body of the Wariri king and contains his soul. During this magical event, a lion cub replaces the maggot and becomes the embodiment of the king (209).

Poikilothermic fish, amphibians, and reptiles are soulless creatures. A striking incident involving an octopus occurs early in the story and is later recalled twice by Henderson. Needing a quiet place to suffer after a fight with Lily, Henderson visits a marine aquarium. He arrives at twilight and an octopus captures his attention:

> The eyes spoke to me coldly. But even more speaking, even more cold, was the soft head with its speckles, a cosmic coldness in which I felt I was dying. The tentacles throbbed and motioned through the glass, the bubbles sped upward, and I thought, "This is my last day. Death is giving me notice." (19)

In Henderson's agitated, emotional state, the cold-blooded stare of the octopus seems innately evil. While descending to the lion's den the first time, Henderson recalls the octopus incident, but realizes he is feeling warmth rather than bone-chilling cold, a sign of a different danger (220). Later when Horko's assistant holds out the shrunken head of a sorceress he claims is a previous incarnation of Atti the lioness, Henderson remembers the sense of " 'This is it! The end!' " he felt upon seeing the octopus.

The frogs Henderson murders in his attempt to purify the Arnewi cistern trouble him. Despite Henderson's obsessive guilt about both the frogs and the now waterless Arnewi, the people are not really much worse off. The water was useless as long as it contained frogs, and draining the cistern was the only ecologi-cally sound way to kill the amphibians. However, whenever Henderson lists his litany of sins, he includes the frogs.

Birds flutter between the pages with surprising regularity and symbolize elation or heightened mood. From night birds to hens, the feathered species and just plain feathers float through religious ceremonies and celebrations. When Dahfu teaches Henderson to roar properly, freeing himself of inhibitions, the king tells his pupil to roar as naturally as birds sing. Dahfu alludes to a piece of writing in which Madam Curie describes "beta particles issuing like flocks of birds" (269). Henderson knows he is no bird and indeed "*would have scared the pterodactyl from the skies*" (284).

Later Henderson echoes the Madam Curie allusion as he describes flocks of birds rising like "masses of notes" (304). Although Romilayu and Henderson suffer hunger in the desert, they manage to eat birds Romilayu kills and once feast on a bird of prey (327).

Ostrich and vulture feathers decorate celebrants during ceremonies, but feathers are also related in one instance to allergy (ceremonies: 146, 176, 180; allergy: 100). Significantly, when Henderson flies out of the wilderness, he dons a hat decorated with feathers in celebration (332–33).

A change in mammal imagery parallels the evolution of the plot. Henderson begins as a pig man and struggles with piggishness, drawing a picture of himself "in pigskin gloves and pigskin shoes, a pigskin wallet in my pocket" (12). Later he envisions his pig self "from the trotters to the helmet, all six feet four inches of me, the picture of that familiar animal, freckled on the belly, with broken tusks and wide cheekbones" (273). The pig image even shares Henderson's dental troubles.

He feels sympathy for the cat he tried to murder and later for the frogs he killed. Cattle trudge thirstily through the Arnewi lands where Henderson first hears of the grun-tu-molani. Despite many mentions, cattle do not figure prominently in the plot. As Dahfu puts it, " 'What could be grun-tu-molani upon a background of cows?' " (269). The Arnewi regard their cows as relatives, but the Wariri sacrifice their cows without sorrow. One interesting mention of cattle refers to Nebuchadnezzar, as Henderson roars "like the great Assyrian bull" (171). Nebuchadnezzar was the "king in Syriac" (Dan. 2.4).

Henderson's drowned brother Dick and King Dahfu are both described as lions. Dahfu's beauty of form is paralleled by a wholeness of soul which Henderson feels as a power emanating from the king. Dahfu represents all that Henderson could be if only he could stop worrying. The big man roars and grows in the power lovingly shared by Dahfu. Because the king is the first person who really understands him, Henderson feels more pain than ever before when Dahfu dies. The king's last request to Henderson is to take care of Atti, but in a plot weakness the lioness disappears from the story. Instead, Henderson takes home the tiny lion cub intended to be Dahfu's reincarnation.

During Henderson's journey home, he recalls another animal— the very first animal who influenced him. As a young man, Henderson worked for a carnival. Smolak, a brown bear, was a "poor broken ruined creature" whom Henderson had been forced to take on the high rides twice daily for the amusement of fair-goers (338). Like Henderson, Smolak had trouble with his teeth. As they clung and cried together on the rides, the bear and Henderson shared love. In reinterpreting this long-buried memory, the big man realizes that if there is little in his nature of true lion-ness, at least he has something of the bear which allows him to roar freely and naturally (336–39).

After braving the lion's den like Daniel, feeling his animal nature like Nebuchadnezzar, and eating locusts like John, Henderson flies toward home with his lion cub and an American orphan who understands only Persian. The big man at last knows what he wants and feels content *being* within his animal nature instead of *becoming* in his unhappy human state. Smolak-like, he cradles the boy in his arms as the bear cradled the younger Henderson. At Newfoundland the plane stops for refueling. Henderson truly is new-found, for he has gained both inner peace and the grun-tu-molani. His problems are not over (Will Lily ever clean up the house? Will he get into medical school?), but he knows how to steer away from the shoals of guilt and grief upon which he has been grounded for so long. Henderson disappears into the white space at the end of the story, running around and around the great silver bird, orphan boy in his arms, "over the frozen ground of almost eternal winter, drawing breaths so deep they shook me, pure happiness" (340).

WORK CITED

Bellow, Saul. *Henderson the Rain King*. New York: Viking, 1967.

"Leaving the Yellow House": Hattie's Will

Walter Shear
Pittsburg State University

In a 1976 interview Saul Bellow concluded, "Unfortunately I just struck the women's movement at a bad time" (Brans 17).[1] Several pieces of evidence tend to support this observation. Not only are there several complaints that Bellow almost exclusively features male protagonists, his few major female characters have seemed, to some irritated readers, to display features which have been labeled typical female weaknesses by those seeking to denigrate, consciously or unconsciously, women. Hattie Wagoner, the leading character of "Leaving the Yellow House," is viewed as a special example. Although two critics, Noriko M. Lippit and Eusebio L. Rodrigues, view Hattie as one of Bellow's survival characters (in Rodrigues' words, "a gnarled, weather-beaten representative of contemporary man" [5]), Constance Rooke's indignant analysis of Hattie still retains some validity. Not only is Hattie a selfish procrastinator, she has none of the ideas or the interest in the intellectual life that ameliorates our condemnation of several of Bellow's similarly weak male protagonists (3).

Few readers would be as moralistically judgmental as Joseph McCadden: Hattie "lacks the mental and physical energy" to arrive at self-knowledge; she is "a wretched failure, responsible for the incoherence of her final days"; and her relationship with Wicks is characterized by "flouting even the minimal standards of civilized conduct in Western society" (214–15). However, even more positive responses to Hattie, such as that of Daniel Fuchs, must struggle with her perverse will. (Fuchs tries to argue that "she transforms the victimization of fate by an irreducible, quixotic narcissism," which succeeds as gesture rather than as deed [296].)

In many respects Hattie's problems are those of the typical Bellow character; indeed, her response to circumstances resembles the weakness and desperation of another character of the same period, Tommy Wilhelm. One of the problems of Bellow's fiction is that while his characters seemingly demand forgiveness from a reader, the author himself remains quite deliberately the intently interested observer, one whose extended analysis of the case seems curiously dependent on his reluctance to finally judge. Although outside the fiction Bellow has said of Hattie simply, "I love her," the narrative conveys no such explicit endorsement (Brans 17).

How can one square Bellow's comment about Hattie with the amount of negative response she has inspired? First, instead of seeing Hattie as representative woman or existential survivor, one ought to place her in the context of Bellow's critique of American culture, specifically in his sorting out of the positive and negative romantic elements in the culture, a concern which culminates in the novel published in 1964, *Herzog*. In doing this, one would not ignore the fact that she is a woman, but would concentrate on what she can do and say because she is a female character.

While Bellow affirms that people must live by something deeper than modern positivism and psychoanalysis (what he refers to as "head culture" [Brans 3]), he also argues that people in Western civilization are foolishly living an extreme romantic individualism in their daily lives without even knowing it: "They think of the proper mode of being as highly stimulated, ecstatic, a life of infinite possibilities, the individual utterly free, his main responsibility to fulfill himself and to realize his desires as richly as he can." For Bellow, the religious perspective is an important key to an alternative mode of thought: "A person finally emerges from all this nonsense when he becomes aware that his life has a much larger meaning he has been ignoring—a transcendent meaning, and that his life is, at its most serious, some kind of religious enterprise, not one that has to do with the hurly-burly of existence" ("Bellow in the Classroom" 976–77).

"Leaving the Yellow House" is a critique of rugged individualism set in what has seemingly become a common context for the idea, the American West. The environment is a harsh desert, a "barren place," with a lake Hattie calls beautiful. Rolfe stresses this country is so isolated only "eccentrics" would want to live in its wilderness. It is a nature whose transcendent evocations provoke frustration rather than contentment for Hattie: "She always ended by looking out of the window at the desert and lake. *They drew you out of yourself. But after they had drawn you, what did they do with you? It was too late to find out. I'll never know. I wasn't meant to*" (33). A prominent part of her first experience in the West was Wicks' defiant interaction with the land. "Wicks had had to shoot their Christmas dinner and she had cooked it—

venison. He killed it on the reservation, and if the Indians had caught them, there would have been hell to pay'' (25). She begins to recognize, especially when Wicks kills (by kicking it to death) the white coyote caught in one of his traps, that this kind of living in nature is savagery. Even with her love of animals, she is forced to accept this level of existence as she embraces Wicks' lifestyle; later when her dog Richie viciously attacks her, she herself kills to survive. She comes to realize that nature here offers no free bounty, that a natural existence may be simply a kind of emptiness, the absence of civilized meaning.

Like Darly, she is not a "genuine" Westerner, but one of the late-comers from the East, and her living in the West seems less a result of a conscious decision than a necessary adaptation to the current facts of her existence: she is without a cent after her divorce; it is Depression time; and Wicks, who knows how to get along in the West, is available. Her pride in her life is connected with her ability to make it through, since as she sees her varied experiences, she concludes, "It has been uphill all the way" (24). It is the Western sense of individuality, especially the independent defiance of convention, that she comes to enjoy, swaggering in her view of Wicks' sexual prowess and of the way the two of them shocked Alice Parmenter. "More than anything else, she wanted to be thought of as a rough, experienced woman of the West" (6). Thus in the hospital she carries on defiantly, swearing almost arrogantly at the nurses.

But while her somewhat silly cheerfulness feeds this notion of herself as an independent survivor, it is primarily an evasion of reality; in point of fact she never despairs completely because she avoids facing the finality of circumstances. Just as the key event of the first half of the story, her accident, remains ambiguously detached from any single explanation (was the significant cause her sneeze, her drunkenness, or was it just chance?), so her independence is propped up throughout the narrative by her uncertainties.

Bellow brings out the depths of both dependence and independence which are stirred because of the inescapable nature of individualism. Part of Hattie's idea of the West links independent character to loyalty and generosity: "People really used to stand by one another in the West" (25). Perhaps inspired by the desperation in her current dependency and weakness (to be unable to drive is to be severely restricted in the contemporary West), she begins to see how often she had acted as the servant in the key relationships in her Western life—with Wicks and with India—and she believes that Pace often took advantage of her as well. While India, we are told, left many scars on her pride, Hattie survived these and received her reward: the house which is at the heart of the narrative. It is, however, the revolt against Wicks' arrogant dominance that is the dramatic climax of the story. Here Hattie's sense of her own dignity—which may be implied elsewhere in the story by her idea of being a "lady"—is suddenly manifested Western-style as she pulls the pistol and says both to Wicks and herself that she has had enough. " '*I couldn't bear to fall so low . . . to be a slave to a shiftless cowboy.*' " Wicks agrees, " 'Guess I went too far. You're right.' " But in looking back, Hattie accuses herself of being too proud and repeats the words India had addressed to her, " 'Forgive me. I hurt myself in my evil' " (40–41).

With the notion of forgiveness—the confession that the self is accountable—Bellow pushes the idea of Western individualism into a religious context of meaning. Hattie, who has been nearly a composite of human weaknesses and careless living, is brought to the point where she accepts the blame for her life. Whereas earlier she had recognized "an idle life was all she was good for" (24), the scriptural overtones of her later accusations—" '*I have taken life. I have lied. I have born false witness. I have stalled*' " (36)—manifest deeper insight. As Rodrigues stresses, "She recognizes the evil within her own self just as she now knows the evil that was present in her dog . . ." (14). This overwhelming sense of weakness leads to dependency on God. However, the fact that Hattie rejects and is repelled by the relentless piety of her brother Angus's household indicates that she is not simply a convert to some old-time religion either.

At this point in the story Hattie's will is not only a literal document determining the heir of her house, it is also her power of decision-making, the primary attribute of her individuality. As she composes, the sense of obligation, of duty to others— especially her family—is mixed with an increasing sense of her significance and insignificance in life. She acknowledges that she does need, if not help, succor—a sign of someone else's genuine concern. She accuses herself of being too proud and of not caring for others as much as she should, of not forgiving enough. Yet in the midst of undermining herself, she comes to know and accept herself in a way she never has before. The act of willing is an absurdity if one believes in it as an absolute act—much as she believes in the modern absolutism of her life as a motion picture from birth. But the importance of willing lies in the fact that it is not simply a critical comment on her, but on her society and on the individualistic philosophy behind that society.

Hattie gets the strongest hint of total significance, not from her death, which is never quite real to her, but from the idea that life is a loan from God. With that concept she can forgive herself: " '*Take what God brings. He gives no gifts unmixed. He makes loans*' " (42). She does not own her life absolutely and she cannot be absolutely responsible. This fits in with her earlier idea: " '*I was never one single thing anyway. . . . Never my own. I was only loaned to myself*' " (33). Yet it also provokes a very human response to want one's own sense of life to count, not simply to be the begging debtor. In willing the yellow house to herself, she is staking a transcendental claim, declaring that the service in her life and the pain of that service (not, she hopes, slavery) is a meaning and can be an honorable identity. One significance is that she has recognized her own worth at least partly.

What Hattie has also discovered in her own helplessness, her own lying fallibility, is the need for human community which an absolute individualism overlooks. For "good" reasons the people around her are not able to respond to such a need. Thus, on an unconscious level, she discovers herself as the one who must recognize and respond to this need. The will, as an objectification of human capacity, suddenly, in a manner both transcendental and irrational, manifests the community which does not exist and, through the offer of impossible help to the undeserving, forgives Hattie for being weakly human.

Here, as elsewhere in Bellow, an idea of being human is tied to a specific cultural situation. The fact that Hattie is a woman allows her to become involved with individualism of the West without being fixated and bound by masculine, macho identity demands. She can seem scandalous in her independence and still move as her physical condition dictates to a dependence that is not tinged with the shameful. Most importantly, she is not inhibited from a spiritual encounter with her weakness as an individual. She has not taken advantage of many of her social opportunities and her pursuit of independence is in several respects shallow, yet from the perspective of her humiliations she senses that her life has some transcendent meaning. That meaning, however, is bound to the weaknesses which inspire it, and in that respect is double-edged. Hattie's story is about her, but about her Western world as well. While Hattie's internal monologue functions to substitute a religious context of meaning for a romantic system of value, her sketched-out flight from institutions and conventions leads to less, not more, freedom, a movement ironically capped by a will which invokes the idea of community only to underline its absence. What survives is not simply Hattie, but her own sense of her being.

NOTE

[1]Specific complaints about Bellow's attitude toward feminism and the female can be found in: Scheffler, Judith. "Two-Dimensional Dynamo: The Female Character in Saul Bellow's Novels." *Wascanna Review* 16.2 (1981): 3–9; Vinoda, Dr. "The Dialectic of Sex in Bellow's Fiction." *Indian Journal of American Studies* 12 (1982): 81–88. For views on the other side see: Aharoni, Ada. "Women in Saul Bellow's Novels." *Studies in American Jewish Literature* 3 (1983): 99–112; Chavkin, Allan. "The Feminism of *The Dean's December*." *Studies in American Jewish Literature* 3 (1983): 113–27.

WORKS CITED

Bellow, Saul. *Mosby's Memoirs and Other Stories*. New York: Viking, 1968. (Contains "Leaving the Yellow House," 1957.)

Brans, Jo. "Common Needs, Common Preoccupations: An Interview with Saul Bellow." *Southwest Review* 62 (1977): 1–19.

Fuchs, Daniel. *Saul Bellow: Vision and Revision*. Durham: Duke UP, 1984.

Lippit, Noriko M. "A Perennial Survivor: Saul Bellow's Heroine in the Desert." *Studies in Short Fiction* 12 (1975): 281–83.

McCadden, Joseph F. *The Flight from Women in the Fiction of Saul Bellow*. Lanham, MD: UP of America, 1980.

Rodrigues, Eusebio L. "A Rough-Hewn Heroine of Our Time: Saul Bellow's 'Leaving the Yellow House.' " *Saul Bellow Journal* 1.1 (1981): 11–17.

Rooke, Constance. "Saul Bellow's 'Leaving the Yellow House': The Trouble with Women." *Studies in Short Fiction* 14 (1977): 184–87.

"Saul Bellow in the Classroom." *College English* 34 (1973): 975–80.

Modern Allegory and the Form of *Seize the Day*

Thomas Loe
SUNY Oswego

Saul Bellow is generally regarded as a realist, but at the same time his characters and their situations are frequently read in terms of the archetypal and symbolic. This is especially true of Bellow's shorter fiction, where the concentrated line of action and sharply focused characters heighten possibilities of metaphoric import. Bellow's shorter works share this characteristic with many others from the modernist period. In fact, a synthesis of the symbolic and the realistic characterizes an increasing number of important narratives in the twentieth century to the point where they may be regarded as a distinct genre. My concern in this essay is to examine *Seize the Day* within the confines of half a dozen major characteristics in the traditional terms of actions, themes, characters, and settings which connect *Seize the Day* with a larger genre. The term I use for addressing *Seize the Day* with this particular focus is modern allegory, which to me seems to be a recognizable type of writing that most generally takes the form of the short novel or novella for twentieth-century fiction. *Seize the Day* seems to be the most appropriate of Bellow's works to deal with in this regard because it is popular and widely taught and because critical views of it have tended to elaborate on both its realistic and metaphoric qualities.

First some definitions. Aside from agreeing about the obviously distinguishing feature of the intermediate length of the novella—somewhere between 15,000 and 50,000 words—most recent interpretations of the form of novellas seem to justify the conclusion that it is the closest thing in modern times we have to allegory. According to Meyer Abrams, allegory is a narrative strategy which may be employed in any literary form or genre "in which the agents and action[s], and sometimes the setting as well, are contrived both to make coherent sense on the 'literal,' or primary level of signification, and also to signify a second, correlated order of agents, concepts, and events" (4). Supporting the notion that the novella resembles allegory are several studies of form that link the novella to other types of illustrative narrative: fable, satire, anatomy or apologue.[1] Graham Good argues that its format "make[s] it more receptive than the novel to communal wisdom, practical guidance, or explicit reflections on the human condition" (210). Perhaps the early twentieth-century concern of making the representative become the illustrative turns the form more decidedly towards the allegorical. In any case, early in the modernist period practitioners of the short novel abandoned the tightly causal plot, balance, spatial unity, and conventionally developed characters of the familiar (perhaps German-dominated) novella. In its place evolved a series of what are regarded as "classics" of the genre written by individuals most closely identified with modernism: Conrad, Joyce, Lawrence, Kafka, Mann, Faulkner, Hemingway, and Fitzgerald. These stories share a remarkable similarity in the external patterns they establish to replace the traditional forms of telling and structuring. A reading of *Seize the Day* in terms of this format establishes that it too should be classified as part of this genre. Because of its restricted and restrained focus, the narrative of the novella is more limited and economical in action, scope, and character than other types of prose fiction. When this is coupled with its philosophically oriented aesthetic intention, it becomes a recognizably distinct genre. Generally these new patterns work thematically to establish a critical distance between their realistic surfaces and their larger, cultural themes.

In aesthetic intention, the novella, like allegory, frequently takes on the foreshortened format resembling those of hypothetical moral or philosophical problems. Because of this purpose, which is intended to enlighten and to illustrate through the working out of some involved ethical issue, the novella can generallly be easily distinguished from other types of prose fiction. The short story and the novel tend to be much more realistic than the novella because the novella's basic impulse is philosophic and metaphoric, not only mimetic. The short story and the novel most generally employ the techniques of verisimilitude. But the novella typically has a single line of action involving a few characters—generally only two or three—only one of whom is developed in depth and whose main concern is self-definition. When these characters are juxtaposed to create the conflict of the plot, they most frequently take on the sort of archetypal triadic arrangement as *Seize the Day* does in its father, son, surrogate-father arrangement. In its tighter, highly selective, chronological frame the shorter length makes more emphatic the restricted series of actions that make short novels appear to be all the more an emblematic crisis or test. We are told that "the particular burden of [Wilhelm's] existence lay upon him like an accretion, a load, a lump" (39). Within the few hours that make up its setting, *Seize the Day* depicts Wilhelm attempting to recapture the "ten such decisions" that make up "the history of his life" (23), much as Marlow in *Heart of Darkness* recaptures in a single story the most formative experience of his life, or Gabriel Conroy in *The Dead* recaptures in the epiphany of a single evening the insight which throws the whole of his prior existence into sharp relief. The novella offers an abstraction, a recapitulation, a distillation of experience: exactly what is being offered in *Seize the Day*.

A chief effect of this retrospective quality of the novella, which is partially created by its attempts to develop a full story simplified in cause and effect through exaggerated, or cataclysmic happenings and choices within a restricted space, is to create a distinctly predetermined cast to the events as they are unfolded (Good 210). In this regard the novella comes to resemble the foregone conclusions frequently present in classical tragedy and is one of the most recognizable elements of the tone and the plot of the genre. Howard Nemerov, for example, develops an extended and eloquent investigation of this in his "Composition and Fate in the Short Novel." Since the major decisions of the protagonist's life have already been made, and the novella is most frequently an attempt to understand why the terms of life have been cast in the mold they seem to take, the end is implicit in the beginning. For this reason it is unusual to find a novella told in optimistic terms where some freedom of control may still exist. So Tommy Wilhelm's "ten such decisions" which determine the direction of his life come to resemble a psychological curse of fate against which he cannot assert his will. But it is primarily the attempt to recapitulate in the brief narrative format some semblance of simplified cause and effect that creates his sense of predetermined failure. Looking at *Seize the Day* within the context of this particular genre reveals that Saul Bellow is no more negative in his presentation of Wilhelm's lack of discipline in this regard than D. H. Lawrence is in his depiction of the fated outcome of the love triangle in *The Fox*, or than Thomas Mann is in his dramatization of Aschenbach's irresistible movement towards death in *Death in Venice*, or than Carson McCuller is in her rendering of love's destructiveness in *The Ballad of the Sad Cafe*.

Most distinct and easily described of the features that distinguish the novella are its patterns of characterization which usually take the form of two juxtaposed or polar individuals. This particular aspect is worth examining in some detail in *Seize the Day*. In the genre one of these personalities is generally realistically developed and sympathetic, the other more distant and metaphoric. One character communicates the confrontation with the real world, especially in terms of surface appearances, the other represents some particular meaningful aspect of that world, a usually hidden, or at least less distinct, aspect better sensed than defined, more elusive and sinister and more connected with the unconscious, the subconscious, the emotional, or the intuitive. Tommy Wilhelm is clearly the former, the mysterious Dr. Tamkin the latter. For the most part the point of view is almost always from the limited and realistic perspective, which enhances the mysterious and metaphoric import of the latter. The elusive, hard-to-articulate symbolic values of, say, Benito Cereno or Mr. Hyde or Leggatt or Kurtz, like those of Dr. Tamkin, are clearly bound up with complex cultural values. Consequently, this sort of juxtaposition is much more explicit than a balanced contrast or simple use of foils would be and allows for the symbolic suggestiveness which links the method of the short novel to that of allegory. The fewer the characters, generally the more emphatic the tie between them. Even though the similarities are not immediately apparent, once their symbolic interdependency is clear they come to represent alter egos or counters of one another.

The importance of this characteristic *Doppelgänger* feature has been emphasized by several critics. Nemerov, for instance, comments on the characters of the short novel: "It is remarkable, too, how often by the device of the double, the incubus as it were, their sufferings and perceptions seem to invade them ambiguously from the world outside and the self within" (239). Dean Flower observes the two central characters are "virtually a shared self" (24). Charles E. May speculates that the predominance of the double in the modern novella "could also be an embodiment of the divided self which R. D. Laing has discussed—a split between the thinking self and the acting self which makes action impossible until the two are integrated" (3293). Many examples of these emblematic juxtapositions abound: the Governess and Peter Quint in *The Turn of the Screw*, Billy Budd and Claggart, Mr. Thompson and Helton in *Noon Wine*, Miss Amelia and Cousin Lymon in *The Ballad of the Sad Cafe*, Nick Carroway and Jay Gatsby, March and Henry in *The Fox*, Tadzio and Aschenbach in *Death in Venice*, and, of course, Tommy Wilhelm and Dr. Tamkin. Dr. Tamkin appears to represent in part the worldliness which both attracts and repels Wilhelm, which he desires and fears, which will save him materially and also destroy his good-natured and naively honest character. In general the kind of juxtaposition provided by the novella allows for a symbolic emphasis that would be undercut if both characters were equally realistic.

This would appear to be the case with Wilhelm and Dr. Tamkin. Wilhelm desires a bond with his father that doesn't exist. In a typically modernist fashion this tie is expressed in terms of money: Wilhelm wishes to receive a demonstration of his father's concern for him by rescuing him from the financial jam he has created for himself. When his father logically but selfishly refuses, Wilhelm intuitively turns instead to "charlatan"-like (96) Tamkin for advice he knows is rationally questionable. In the same manner he had earlier intuitively turned away from college— supposedly a source of rational learning—to the sympathetic bonds offered by the questionable talent scout Maurice Venice, later revealed as another charlatan, even though Wilhelm realizes Venice cast him as a loser from the beginning. Why? Typically in the novella this sort of empathetic bonding that takes place— between secret sharers of oppositie inclinations like Marlow and Kurtz or Jekyll and Hyde—puts the innocent in the hands of the more experienced self. The kind of *Doppelgänger* intuitiveness that links Wilhelm to Dr. Tamkin works to destroy innocence (as it does in other novellas) in terms of its own modern reality, financial success. This metaphorical separation allows for allegorical dramatizing of the destruction of the different aspects of self. The pattern is reconfirmed emphatically at the conclusion of *Seize the Day* when Wilhelm instinctively turns in at a funeral to mourn the destruction of a metaphorical aspect of himself. It also explains Dr. Tamkin's lecture on the two souls battling against each other. It makes sense of why Wilhelm is given so many different names—Wilhelm, Tommy, Wilky, Velvel. One could argue, too, that typically this process of partial self-destruction leads to epiphanic insight, like that given through the vicarious bonding of Miranda with the dead Adam Barclay in *Pale Horse, Pale Rider*, even though that insight may lead only to a crippling impotency.

Frequently, modern novellas utilize their narrators as vehicles for undertaking a journey to understand the nature of truth itself, and their self-consciousness in relating their experiences allows for a complication of perspective that qualifies and makes ironic their discoveries. So, even though we think of allegory as a strategy that typically operates within established standards of belief, the novella is a way of using the methods of allegory to explore the nature of truth when there is no generally accepted truth to be offered. This Zen-like paradox finds a perfect avenue for its perspective in the koan-like riddles complicated by point of view in *Seize the Day*. Perhaps Wilhelm is described as having a "Buddha's Head" (82) and Dr. Tamkin "pagoda like" shoulders (62) in order to reinforce the sense of this paradox. The changes in perspectives in the story, which is told not only from Wilhelm's point of view, but also from Dr. Adler's (27, 36, 42, 54), and even from Rubin's (15) and the Estonian woman's (106), offer ironic layering and distancing imposssible to achieve by a consistent and more realistic single perspective. Similarly, the unreliable narrator of *The Turn of the Screw*, or the growing awareness of a naive perspective such as that revealed in *The Aspern Papers*, or the "second person" perspective of *The Great Gatsby*, or the "detached" but dramatized view of *Daisy Miller*, or the parable-like rendering of *Innocent Erêndira* allows for both intimacy and distance, a relation of events and, at the same time, a creation of uncertainty of what exactly has happened. This multiplicity of self-conscious "framing" (Good 210) for narrative is certainly not unique to the short novel, but the concise format of the short novel makes it much more likely that its audience will retain a more complete sense of the focus of events. This may account for its frequency as a complicating feature inherent in the novella's point of view. The modernistic tendency to take a comic perspective as one way of dealing with an absurd reality also allows for a simultaneous distancing and intimacy that is characteristic not only of *Seize the Day*, but of Bellow's fiction in general (Cohen 95).

The typical short length, single line of action, metaphoric setting, and unified thematic focus of the short novel allow for the possibility of subtle exploration of values through ironic and shifting perspective; modern practitioners of the novella quickly realized its potential for exploring the elusive standards of their time. One need only compare the authoritative focus established by the point of view in eighteenth-century novellas like *Candide* or *Rasselas* to the inscrutable open-endedness of more comtemporary novellas like *Seize the Day* to establish clearly that point of view as utilized by the modernistic short novel can become an ideal medium for reexamining values.

An allegorical thrust also affects the structure and setting of a work, and in the novella the usual result is a journey or quest. Frequent application of terms like *Bildungsroman* or picaresque (Nault) to Saul Bellow's fiction is particularly appropriate within this context. In spite of its mimetic surface, the modernistic novella has the sorts of symbolic patterns that frequently result in its becoming the fable of the search for identity. Almost regardless of the mimetic social surroundings that work to establish its level of realism, many short novels follow some fairly well-defined patterns of action, what might almost be called ritualistic patterns, generally within an intensified, concentrated setting. Flower, for example, feels setting is so important to the short novel that it takes on the force of a personality and is frequently aligned in a triadic arrangement with the other juxtaposed characters (13–26). This appears to me to generate most often the major conflict in short novels. Setting and plot are intricately bound up with each other in short novels in so intense a fashion that no other narrative, besides that of traditional allegory, resembles them. The very brevity of short novels tends to focus attention on the possibility of significance in every detail, and it is this brevity which allows the setting to be made unique and believable, and at the same time metaphorical.

In establishing the setting of the dreary alienation of New York City, which we are told is "the end of the world" (83), and in drawing parallels with Edmund Spenser's quest themes by using pointed references to Hotel Gloriana, *Seize the Day* again resembles other modern novellas. *Heart of Darkness* is another important example of a novella in which the setting is established in sparse, concentrated, impressionistic strokes that seem to lend layers of possible interpretation to every detail and image. Likewise, *Death in Venice* works to accumulate the effects of death and decay. Within these intensified settings the conflicts that evolve are, again, both intimate and distanced, closely resembling the loosely jointed and episodic actions of the *Bildungsroman*. Consequently, they de-emphasize causality and emphasize the symbolic suggestiveness of the mysterious signs associated with ritual initiation. Wilhelm, for instance, "rejected [the] begging and denied the omen" of the "hoary old fiddler" (105) who ominously points his bow at him when he finally leaves the brokeage office after the descent of his fortunes. Even more obvious are Dr. Adler's expletives invoking the name of Christ during Wilhelm's last confrontation with him. These help establish other parallels with archetypal descent. Clearly these allegorical quest motifs help unify the story on a thematic level.

In this regard, one of the most commonly repeated striking structural patterns in the modern novella is the archetypal cycle of symbolic immersion with death and a following rebirth. Most frequently, the less realistic, but more symbolic "double" is the one who undergoes the direct experience with death; the more realistic partner—the more empathetic character from whom the point of view comes—is the one who remains behind, "alive" but symbolically afflicted because of the strong identification with the "other." The modern preoccupation with the themes of sterility and impotence is especially well served by this allegorical conflict of sublimated or vicarious experience through these sorts of sympathetic identifications because the knowledge gained through such an experience typically renders the main protagonist incapable of action. Having had one's innocent idealism destroyed in such fashion frequently creates an embittered or cynical or futile environment where further struggle appears useless.

A surprisingly wide range and number of modern novellas conclude with such a life-to-death-to-rebirth cycle, probably because it is an almost ideal way to combine the mimetic and metaphoric, to synthesize the two levels necessary to allegory into a sense of resolution, without becoming blatantly obvious in its symbolism (Springer 20–25). Looking at such works with a sense of the genre's larger narrative tradition allows for a recognition of such a cycle that might otherwise be obscured. Especially because themes associated with modernism tend to be negative (*Seize the Day* not untypically uses "morbid guilt," "cripple," "sickening," "curse," and "impotent" [97] in the course of two sentences), lessons of qualified optimism that do appear may easily remain cryptic and concealed without such a perspective. The epilogue-like final actions common to novellas consist of the rebirth part of the cycle and should be seen at least as a stoic or comic awareness of fate rather than a passive indifference to it or an unrealistically naive perception of it. This is most clear, for instance, in a novella like *The Dead* where Gabriel Conroy redefines himself through his metaphorical identification with Michael Furey and the rest of humanity in the "generous tears" (681) that cloud his vision at the moment of his epiphanic experience.

This rebirth continuum exists less obviously, but is more important to note for that reason, in something like the seemingly gratuitous identification that Wilhelm makes with the dead man whose funeral he stumbles into at the end of *Seize the Day*, and which seems to incapacitate Wilhelm from further action. The novella begins on the first page with his descent in the elevator and, as critics like M. Gilbert Porter have meticulously demonstrated, follows through with pervasive water imagery leading to the underground pool and Wilhelm's final submergence "beneath the wat'ry floor" (13) in the release of his "quelled tears" (56) in the "happy oblivion of tears" (118) of the final scene. Presenting sublimated deaths in such ritualistic fashion seemingly allows the catharsis necessary for rebirth. Portraying archetypal cycles in this manner perserves the story's realism and allows for a commentary on the moral precepts being entertained. It seems to be a happy compromise between straightforward exposition and dramatic representation which is exactly the strength of the novella.

Approaching *Seize the Day* in this manner is useful because it helps establish some notion of the continuity that exists between it and many of the novellas of very disparate writers like Evelyn Waugh, Conrad, Joyce, Lawrence, Kafka, Faulkner, McCullers, and Mann—only some could be mentioned in the scope of this essay. The perspective of this larger tradition of form should help reveal how Bellow realistically and convincingly utilizes recognizable patterns designed to reflect the depth and complexity of psychic involvement necessary for dealing with the tensions of modern life. When an understanding of allegory as a method of communicating abstract concepts is combined with an understanding of modernism and the form of the novella, we should understand all the better one of the important avenues of expression for the present creative imagination. Through this form Bellow provides a structure for examining and exposing the frailties of the defenses established to protect against those tensions, and he provides a sense of movement and of ending, without unrealistically resolving the ambiguities generated by those tensions.

NOTE

For studies linking the novella to other types of illustrative narrative, see Richter 12, Scholes 108, Frye 311, Springer 10, and Leibowitz 78.

WORKS CITED

Abrams, M. H. *A Glossary of Literary Terms*. 4th ed. New York: Holt, 1981.

Bellow, Saul. *Seize the Day*. New York: Viking, 1976.

Cohen, Sarah Blacher. *Saul Bellow's Enigmatic Laughter*. Urbana: U of Illinois P, 1974.

Flower, Dean S. Introduction. *Eight Short Novels*. Ed. Dean S. Flower. Greenwich, CT: Fawcett, 1967.

Frye, Northrup. *Anatomy of Criticism*. Princeton: Princeton UP, 1957.

Good, Graham. "Notes on the Novella." *Novel* 10 (1977): 197–211.

Harper, Gordon Lloyd. "Saul Bellow." *Writers at Work: The Paris Review Interviews*, Third Series. 1967. Rpt. in *Saul Bellow: A Collection of Critical Essays*. Ed. Earl Rovit. Englewood Cliffs: Prentice, 1975. 5–18.

Joyce, James. "The Dead." *Reading Modern Short Stories*. Palo Alto: Scott, 1955.

Leibowitz, Judith. *Narrative Purpose in the Novella*. The Hague: Mouton, 1974.

May, Charles E. "The Novella." *Critical Survey of Long Fiction*. English Language Series. Vol. 8. Ed. Frank N. Magill. Englewood Cliffs: Salem Press, 1983. 3213–3352.

Nault, Marianne. *Saul Bellow: His Works and His Critics: An Annotated International Bibliography*. New York: Garland, 1977.

Nemerov, Howard. "Composition and Fate in the Short Novel." *The Graduate Journal* 5 (1963). Rpt. in *Poetry and Fiction: Essays*. New Brunswick: Rutgers UP, 1963. 229–45.

Porter, M. Gilbert. "The Scene as Image: A Reading of *Seize the Day*." *Saul Bellow: A Collection of Critical Essays*. Ed. Earl Rovit. Englewood Cliffs: Prentice, 1975. 52–71.

Richter, David. Introduction. *Forms of the Novella: Ten Short Novels*. Ed. David Richter. New York: Knopf, 1981.

Scholes, Robert and Robert Kellogg. *The Nature of Narrative*. New York: Oxford UP, 1966.

Springer, Mary Doyle. *Forms of the Modern Novella*. Chicago: U of Chicago P, 1975.

Book Reviews

A Book Review of *Saul Bellow: An Annotated Bibliography, Second Edition* by Gloria L. Cronin and Blaine H. Hall. New York: Garland Publishing. 1987. 312 pp.

Those interested in Bellow's work will certainly welcome the publication of this excellent new bibliography. In 1977 Garland published Marianne Nault's *Saul Bellow: His Works and His Critics: An Annotated International Bibliography*, but it contained a distressing number of errors and suffered from poor organization. Nault listed the criticism on Bellow's work alphabetically by author, and this feature and an inadequate index made it impossible to quickly find criticism on a particular novel, short story, or play. I suspect that in place of Nault's bibliography, many people used Leslie Field and John Z. Guzlowski's "Criticism of Saul Bellow: A Selected Checklist," in *Modern Fiction Studies*, for Field and Guzlowski list criticism in a logical way with sections on each of the novels.

In contrast to Nault's book, Cronin and Hall organize their bibliography in an effective manner. There is a clearly written introduction that explains the organization and rationale of their book. The authors divide the section on primary sources into these categories: novels, short fiction, plays, essays, miscellaneous writings, and interviews. The section on secondary sources includes subdivisions on bibliographies and checklists, books and monographs, special journal issues, biographical sources, doctoral dissertations, and criticism and reviews. The section on criticism and reviews includes subdivisions on "General Articles, Chapters, and Reviews," "Plays," "Short Fiction," "To Jerusalem and Back," and each of Bellow's novels.

Cronin and Hall wisely do not include everything Bellow has published nor everything published on his work. They do not include some early short publications later published in longer works. (These short publications can be found in Nault's bibliography for those scholars who are interested in investigating the extent of Bellow's revising of his published work.) They omit early critical reactions and sketchy reviews, but they do include and often annotate articles and reviews with substantive critical analysis.

Cronin and Hall also made a sensible decision on their approach to annotations, which are usually descriptive and only occasionally evaluative. They do indicate the major articles, however, and this information will be welcomed by students of Bellow's work who may feel overwhelmed with the amount of scholarship before them. There are, for example, 150 articles and reviews just on *Herzog*.

When I consider the enormous amount of work the authors put into this impressive book, I hesitate to suggest changes for a future bibliography. But there are some things I would have done differently. The authors chose not to annotate books. I would not only annotate books but also evaluate them. For example, readers would find it useful to know that Daniel Fuchs' *Saul Bellow: Vision and Revision* is one of the best books on Bellow and that Fuchs brilliantly analyzes Bellow's process of composition. He spent more than a decade transcribing and studying Bellow's vast manuscript collection, a Herculean task, for there are more than four thousand manuscript pages on even a relatively straightforward novel such as *Henderson the Rain King*. It would be useful, too, for the reader to know that Jan Bakker in his book *Fiction as Survival Strategy: A Comparative Study of the Major Works of Ernest Hemingway and Saul Bellow* did not demonstrate that he is aware that Bellow has commented on Hemingway's fiction in his interviews, reviews, and essays, and that Hemingway read and liked Bellow's early works. In their superb selective bibliography, "Saul Bellow" (in *American Novelists*, volume one of *Contemporary Authors Bibliographical Series* [Detroit: Gale, 1986, 83–155]), Cronin and Liela H. Goldman do summarize and evaluate books on Bellow, and I suspect that Cronin and Hall did not feel it was necessary to repeat this information in their bibliography. Nevertheless, I think it would be useful to have this information in the standard bibliography of Bellow.

It would be useful, too, if Cronin and Hall included some brief annotations in the section on bibliographies and checklists and indicate what, if anything, is still valuable about each one of them. They might mention, for example, that even Nault's bibliography, despite its shortcomings, has two features that may be useful to some people. In addition to listing Bellow's short fiction that later became parts of novels, Nault also presents information on Bellow's manuscript collections at the University of Chicago, though Cronin and Hall note that Nault's information is "incomplete and inaccurate" because manuscript material has been added and the collection has been rearranged. Cronin and Hall do not include information on Bellow's manuscript collections because "the major repositories of Bellow's materials have limited access," invariably requiring Bellow's permission.

I would also urge the authors to include in the next edition of the bibliography a separate category for audio-visual materials. There are several audiotapes of Bellow expressing his ideas, a Caedmon audiotape of Bellow reading excerpts from *Herzog*, a videotape of *Seize the Day*, an excellent unabridged recording of *Mosby's Memoirs and Other Stories* (by Books on Tape), as well as other items. One could argue that a listing of audio-visual materials is not typically found in bibliographies, but, in any case, such a listing is useful.

These changes that I have offered for the next edition of the Bellow bibliography are not major ones, and there is no question that Cronin and Hall's distinguished bibliography easily surpasses all other bibliographies on Bellow's work. Its index includes not only names and works but also subjects (e.g., Anti-Semitism; production history) and is more useful than the indexes of other bibliographies. Cronin and Hall's annotations are better than those in other bibliographies. Most important, this bibliography includes more information on Bellow's work than any other. Two examples will support this claim. In the section on interviews, Cronin and Hall list about a dozen more interviews than Nault does for the same period of time. In the absence of a biography of Bellow, one especially appreciates Cronin and Hall's section entitled "Biographical Sources," which lists almost three dozen items. No other bibliography provides the reader with this kind of information. In short, scholars and serious students of Bellow's work owe an enormous debt to Cronin and Hall for collecting, and often annotating, the 1388 entries in their bibliography.

Allan Chavkin
Southwest Texas State University

A Book Review of *More Die of Heartbreak* by Saul Bellow. New York: William Morrow Co., 1987. 335 pp.

Those acquainted with the family of Saul Bellow novels will immediately recognize family resemblances in the latest addition to that group, *More Die of Heartbreak*. The narrator acknowledges his "weakness for the big issues," such things as the fate of man in the modern world and the meaning of human love. He is one of those familiar Bellow theorizers who combine the perceptive and the preposterous, the wise and the wacky. His discourse spans the distance from the abstract niceties of Hegelian philosophy to the particular sordid intricacies of graft in machine politics. Within this discourse, sophisticated literary and philosophic allusions rub shoulders with the colloquial and slangy. It's like a buzzing cocktail party where you are as likely to run into William Blake as Ronald McDonald. The novel focuses on the familiar Bellow situation of the intelligent man totally inept and victimized in his relationships with women; as usual, this situation is part of the larger one of the simple-hearted man among the Machiavellians. The narrator is concerned with the "spiritual headaches" caused by present-day American society, for which people take the nostrum of "sexual Tylenol."

These are some of the family traits. Another one, which has become increasingly prominent in Bellow's later novels, is a preoccupation with the transcendent, with the aspects of human experience and the qualities of the human soul that lie beyond the purview of positivistic science and psychology or rationalistic philosophy. And it is this preoccupation, above all others, that provides the active principle for *More Die of Heartbreak*. It is a religious preoccupation, if a broad definition of religion is allowed. In fact, this statement from Hume's *Dialogues Concerning Natural Religion* seems to illuminate the method and effect of this novel:

> I am indeed persuaded, said Philo, that the best and indeed
> the only method of bringing every one to a due sense of
> religion, is by just representations of the misery and wicked-
> ness of men. And for that purpose a talent of eloquence
> and strong imagery is more requisite than that of reasoning

and argument. For is it necessary to prove what every one feels within himself? 'Tis only necessary to make us feel it, if possible, more intimately and sensibly.

Bellow's eloquent images (the eloquence heightened by his comic vision) do indeed acquaint us intimately and sensibly with the misery and wickedness in contemporary life. And while the novel contains a good deal of reasoning and argument, this intellectualizing actually functions as part of the images. As the narrator admits, "these cognitive efforts will never get us anywhere." In fact, in this portrait of contemporary life, excessive rationalism is a principal source of the misery and wickedness. "A sense of religion" is a suitable phrase for describing the effect of this novel if emphasis on the transcendent in the human soul and on the importance of efficacious love are considered central to the religious sense.

The narrator, Kenneth Trachtenberg, is a 35-year-old assistant professor of Russian literature at a university in the Midwest's rustbelt. Having grown up in Paris, he has come to America in a spirit of quest to be near his uncle, Benn Crader, a distinguished botonist who teaches at the same university. In Kenneth's estimation, Benn is "one of those passionate natures who long to find and see what perhaps does not exist on earth." He has charisma, or what Kenneth calls "magics." As a "plant mystic" he uses plants as his arcana—what you need to know "to prepare for the communication of spiritual mystery." Kenneth considers Benn a "Citizen of Eternity," fellow citizen (although perhaps well down the scale or even in the process of naturalization) with the great prophets and sublime artists. Unfortunately, Benn's gifts for contemplation and unselfish love do not suit him for confronting contempoary life and particularly contemporary women. He is "a woman-battered man"—"a visionary with plants, a dub with women." Therefore, Kenneth has come to learn a kind of mystic wisdom from him and at the same time protect him from sexual entanglements. In this mutually dependent relationship, Ken believes they have a "crucial project" going: to bring to human life the visionary gifts Benn brought to plant life, "to transpose his magical powers from botany to love."

In leaving Paris, Kenneth rejected French intellectualism and his father's talented and obsessive womanizing. Neither, he thinks, can teach him to be a Citizen of Eternity. The former, in its abstraction, is out of touch with the mystery of human personality adhering in concrete experience; the latter is "death-flavored."

But the novel's comic irony derives from his being himself an inveterate and quirky intellectual theorizer and a vulnerable bumbler with women. Thus, the book provides variations of two characteristic Bellow paradigms. The first is the paradoxical situation of a cerebral author creating a cerebral character who provides a cerebral critique of cerebral activity. The second is the situation of the intellectual male with a rational and slightly misogynistic perception of female entanglements who nevertheless is a sucker for them.

Kenneth's contradictory philosophic urges derive from two contrasting influences absorbed during his youth in Paris. One was the philosopher Alexandre Kojève—"a relentless, merciless reasoner"—who occasionally took dinner in his parents' home. (Kojève, an actual person, gave an important series of lectures in Paris during the thirties on the philosophy of Hegel and consequently influenced French philosophy since that time.) Kenneth traces his weakness for "the big overview" back to him. The second influence was his first Russian language teacher, M. Yermelov, a student of the mystical tradition who propounded the notion that each of us has an angel, "a being charged with preparing us for a higher evolution of the spirit" and instilling warmth into our souls. Yermelov warned him "against the glamour of thought, the calculating intellect and its constructions, its fabrications alien to the power of life." These influences represent highly rationalistic philosophy on the one hand and mystical wisdom of the heart on the other. Bellow, drawing upon cabalistic writing and widening the implications of Benn's botany, uses the terms Tree of Knowledge and Tree of Life to identify these opposing impulses. The Tree of Knowledge is associated in this context with the truth of striving, with calculated power concerns in the areas of money, politics, technology, and sex. The Tree of Life is linked with the truth of receptivity, with love, family bonds, and the transcendent concerns of Swedenborg, Blake, and a cluster of Russian mystic philosophers (Berdyaev is among them, and the novel bears the stamp of his philosophy). According to Yermelov, "knowledge divorced from life equals sickness." The condition of contemporary America is symbolically epitomized by the fact that the book treating the Tree of Life is buried at the site of Benn's family family home under the Electronic Tower, a skyscraper built by another of Kenneth's uncles, who is the very embodiment of greed and political corruption.

According to cabalistic tradition, the Tree of Knowledge and the Tree of Life would eventually unite. The need for such union is reflected in Kenneth's acknowledgment that skyscrapers, though filled with "abominable enterprises," do "express an aspiration for freedom, a rising above," and, perhaps deceptively, "transmit an idea of transcendence." Moreover, while recognizing the advantages of living in isolation from a time in which the Tree of Knowledge dominates (Benn's apartment is described as a "defense system" against contemporary urban society), Kenneth knows such escape is neither possible nor desirable: "When you come down into contemporary life, you can really get it in the neck. If on the other hand you decline to come down into it, you'll never understand a *thing*." Behind Kenneth's words is Bellow's understanding that the good that emerges from a conflict of values arises not from the total abandonment or destruction of one set of values but from the building of a new value, sustained, like an arch, by the tension of the original two. But such a new value will never be achieved without what Kenneth frequently refers to as "a turning point" for humankind, which begins as a turning point in the individual, usually in individuals assigned to the humanities, "the nursery games of humankind, which had to be left behind when the age of science began." Such a turning point will be the product of love. Kenneth quotes Philip Larkin: "In everyone there sleeps a sense of life according to love." The problem at present, he adds, is that the "rationally wicked" are the more wide awake.

The novel is rich in recurring motifs subtley interwoven to develop the theme suggested in the title. An aggressive newspaperman comes to Benn for a statement about plant life and the increasing levels of radiation and toxic wastes. " 'It's terribly serious, of course,' " Benn finally responds, " 'but I think more people die of heartbreak than of radiation.' " In other words, the threats posed to heart and soul—our spiritual nature—by the contemporary world outweigh in importance the threats to our physical existence. The narrator repeatedly chafes (as did Swedenborg, who is mentioned over a dozen times) at the conception of nature as an enclosed prison, "a fixed world of matter and energy." He refers to this mechanistic interpretation as the "literal" view and observes that "the interest in human beings is quickly exhausted by literalness." "To be seen literally," he says, "dries out one's humanity." And this literalness is particularly lethal from a sexual standpoint because, taken literally, sexual relations, which should be a manifestation of love *par excellence*, become diminished and degraded and "Eros faces annihilation." On the other hand, "by pushing to the very borders of literalness you got into visionary areas which science wanted nothing to do with." It is the visionary areas that fascinate the narrator.

His quest for the visionary areas is comic. Bellow, like his narrator, has "a weakness for the big issues," but he never treats the search for ultimate answers without the leaven of irony and parody. Henderson's quest is a notable example in this regard. Kenneth is delightfully ridiculous in his rationalistic attacks on rationalism. By his own admission he is "a bit on the weird side and notorious for the kinkiness of my theories." Much of the comedy in this novel originates in the "gap between high achievement and personal ineptitude." "The greater your achievements, the less satisfactory your personal and domestic life will be." Kenneth asks in exasperation, "Why was it necessary for the Father of Cybernetics to have his zipper checked by his wife before he left the house?" And of course tuning in to the visionary areas particularly puts one out of sync with mundane affairs. The attempt to live in a higher world of mystery, love, and soul, while at the same time trying to confront domestic, financial, technological, political, and especially sexual problems, is a fertile source of comedy. Being a Citizen of Eternity doesn't prevent one from being a fool and may even assure it.

Treating the big issues with comedy and irony and putting his own convictions in the mouths of characters who are quirky and often preposterous has allowed Bellow over the years to insinuate his ideas and values without having to be directly accountable for them to a critical audience that would readily attack them if they were openly asserted. His novels have secrets, as people do. They are there as a bonus for the sensitive reader or as a kind of subliminal quavering. Some view his technique as overly cagey or even cowardly, but whether that was ever true or not, it does not seem to apply to his later work, which has become increasingly explicit in its concern with transcendence. And consider this statement from his preface to Allan Bloom's *The Closing of the American Mind*:

> But the channel [to the soul] is always there, and it is our business
> to keep it open, to have access to the deepest parts of ourselves—
> to that part of us which is conscious of a higher consciousness, by
> means of which, we make final judgments and put everything

together. The independence of this consciousness, which has the strength to be immune to the noise of history and the distractions of our immediate surroundings, is what the life struggle is all about. The soul has to find and hold its ground against hostile forces, sometimes embodied in ideas which frequently deny its very existence and which indeed often seem to be trying to annul it altogether.

This statement, which accurately describes the central concern of *More Die of Heartbreak*, very openly reveals his deepest convictions.

A more adequate explanation for why Bellow puts wisdom in the mouths of preposterous characters and why his seekers for the big truths are always inept in the little truths of ordinary affairs lies in his lively awareness that, given the nature of mortal existence, wisdom is inevitably and inextricably mixed with folly, the sublime is never distant from the ridiculous, and the most inspired seer is ineluctably alloyed with a generous amount of human klutziness. In Bellow's view, it is an error, on the one hand, to deny the existence of the big truths, and on the other, to think any human will ever express them purely and definitively, let alone incorporate them into daily behavior. It is best to treasure the fragments and intimations wherever we find them in the poignant comedy of modern life.

As usual, Bellow's critique of modern life in this novel is wide ranging, from the large issues of East–West relations to the quality of frozen dinners. But his special concern is with what Yermelov calls "intellect without soul." The narrator describes this as "the classic modern challenge" and repeatedly emphasizes that hyperactive but unfocused consciousness is the cause of our decline. "The tom-toms beating inside our heads, driving us crazy, are the Great Ideas." We prize as insight "the restlessness or oscillation of modern consciousness." It takes the place of prayer for us. But "these proliferating thoughts have more affinity to insomnia than to mental progress. Oscillations of the mental substance is what they are, ever-increasing jitters." They won't be overcome by calculation, but only by "a power of life." Near the end of his story, the narrator concludes:

> The secret of our being still asks to be unfolded. Only now we understand that worrying at it and ragging it is no use. The first step is to stop these oscillations of consciousness that are keeping me awake. Only, before you command the oscillations to stop, before you check out, you must maneuver yourself into a position in which metaphysical aid can approach.

What he means by "metaphysical aid" is a subject for speculation. One thing is certain: Bellow, through eloquence and strong images, does bring us to a sense of religion, and he does it more entertainingly and provocatively than does any other current American novelist.

Stephen L. Tanner
Brigham Young University

A Book Review on *Le génocide dans la fiction romanesque* by Charlotte Wardi. Presses Universitaires de France, 1986. 179 pp. 95FF.

Forty years after the full extent and horror of the Holocaust was recognized, the question of its literary representation remains a vexed one. To paraphrase Elie Wiesel, either a novel about Auschwitz is not a novel, or it is not about Auschwitz. Charlotte Wardi's recent study (in French) situates the representation of genocide in a more general context of ethical and aesthetic questions, investigating the problematic relation between history and fiction, the real and the imagined. About half of the book considers such problems as the choice of a fictional form adequate to the subject of the Holocaust, the creation of character, the use of language, and the different perspectives of writer–survivors as opposed to writers without direct historical experience.

Throughout the book, the author (herself a survivor) writes with an informed sense of the debates which the subject has occasioned, providing a careful consideration of the major issues. Thus, the difficulties posed by the individualistic bias of the novel, which militates against an authentic rendering of collective experience, are reviewed, and the author also tackles the problem of form, considering whether the insertion of a profoundly irrational event into an ordered structure may tend in some sense to justify the completely unjustifiable, rationalizing the unreasonable. Thereafter, Wardi adopts a comparative approach, discussing novels by Bellow, Romain Gary, Heinrich Böll, and William Styron, writers from quite distinct backgrounds, who propose different fictive solutions.

In contrast to Gary, whose knowledge of Judaism appears somewhat superficial, Wardi highlights the extent to which Bellow is firmly rooted in Jewish culture, proceeding to consider the more problematic positions of Böll, as a Catholic and anti-Nazi, and Styron, who is seen as employing Auschwitz largely as an illustration of his views on slavery. (Styron comes off very much the worst in the comparison.) On the whole the discussion of *Mr. Sammler's Planet* rarely rises above the level of intelligent plot-summary, simplifying the novel in thematic terms. The black pickpocket, for example, becomes nothing more than a force of nature, with a consequent underestimation of the complexity of Bellow's investigation of the opposition between nature and culture. There are also one or two unfortunate typos. (Mr. Sammler becomes "Slammer" on one occasion.)

The overall point, treated by Bellow in common with Gary— that genocide is the starting point for a philosophical reflection on the nature of history and of society—is firmly substantiated. Bellow's strategy, extending from the Holocaust to question the whole Western conception of man and of his world, is particularly appropriate. To quote Wiesel once more, "At Auschwitz, not only man died, but the idea of man."

Judie Newman
University of Newcastle upon Tyne

Selected Annotated Critical Bibliography for 1986

Gloria L. Cronin
Blaine H. Hall
Brigham Young University

Articles and Chapters

Alter, Robert. "Kafka's Father, Agnon's Mother, Bellow's Cousins." *Commentary* Feb. 1986: 46–52.

Provides a general discussion of the family in fiction, proceeds to the Jewish family depicted in America in Jewish fiction, and provides a pointed discussion of how families in Bellow's fiction are usually extended rather than nuclear families. Claims that "the Jewish immigrant extended family draws him [Bellow] because it offers such a splendid sampling of human variety, and it is the extravagant particularity of individual character that engages him." Concentrates primarily on the short story "Cousins" which, Alter argues, takes the definition of "cousins" to embrace humanity at large.

Anderson, David D. "The Novelist as Playwright: Saul Bellow on Broadway." *Saul Bellow Journal* 5.1 (1986): 48–62.

Reviews briefly Bellow's history of involvement with the theater and his writings both for it and about it. Discusses several dramatic pieces including "The Wrecker" and *The Last Analysis*. Discusses the textual evolution of *LA* and the character of Bummidge. Concludes with Bellow's responses concerning his broadway career.

Bach, Gerhard. "Saul Bellow's German Reception. Part I." *Saul Bellow Journal* 5.2 (1986): 52–65.

Describes in considerable detail American writers and postwar Germany, Bellow publications in German, German readers and reviewers, German critics, and the German position. A major article. Part II is scheduled for publication in *SBJ* 6.1 (1987).

Berger, Alan L. "Holocaust Survivors in *Anya* and *Mr. Sammler's Planet*." *Modern Language Studies* 16.1 (1986): 81–87.

Deals with the psycho-social catastrophe of the Holocaust as Berger traces the Holocaustal reactions of Anya, Ninka, Shula and Mr. Sammler in terms of survivor missions to clarify identity and recreate a moral universe.

Bouson, J. Brooks. "The Narcissistic Self-Drama of Wilhelm Adler: A Kohutian Reading of Bellow's *Seize the Day*." *Saul Bellow Journal* 5.2 (1986): 3–14.

Bellow, through his character Wilhelm Adler, anticipates recent psychoanalytic investigations into the dynamics of the narcissistic personality disorder. Wilhelm Adler provides an artistic anticipation of what psychoanalyst Heinz Kohut describes as "tragic," "broken" man, the narcissistically defective individual "who suffers from an enfeebled, crumbling sense of self."

Brackenhoff, Mary. "*Humboldt's Gift*: The Ego's Mirror—A Vehicle for Self-Realization." *Saul Bellow Journal* 5.2 (1986): 15–21.

Discusses the fact that his protagonists are frequently blinded "by their egocentricity [and] need to distance themselves from their own strong personalities in order to examine and, hopefully, redirect their lives. To aid his protagonists Bellow has frequently employed a narrative ingenuity or cast of secondary characters to provide mirror images, alter egos, or reality instructors—points of view that throw the protagonists' characters into relief."

Bradbury, Malcolm. " 'The Nightmare in Which I am Trying to Get a Good Night's Rest': Saul Bellow and Changing

History." Ed. Edmond Schraepan. Brussels: Centrum Voor Taal En Literatuuwetenschap, Vrije Universiteit Brussel, 1978. Symposium held at the Free University of Brussels (V.U.B.) on 10–11 Dec. 1977. Rpt. in *Saul Bellow*. Ed. Harold Bloom. Modern Critical Views. New York: Chelsea, 1986. 129–46.

Attempts to account for dark places in the novels and to detail Bellow's European appeal. Discusses also the ambiguous Bellow ending in light of the themes of darkness and the influence of European thinking in the novels and concludes that the Bellow hero lives in a world where metaphysical measurements cannot be taken and yet where the mind insists that they be taken anyway.

Chase, Richard. "The Adventures of Saul Bellow: Progress of a Novelist." *Commentary* 27.4 (1959): 323–30. Rpt. in *Saul Bellow and the Critics*. Ed. Irving Malin. New York: New York UP, 1967. 25–38; *Saul Bellow*. Ed. Harold Bloom. Modern Critical Views. New York: Chelsea, 1986. 13–24.

A general discussion of a variety of aspects of the novel. Primarily a first response review article. Many fruitful ideas mentioned but not developed. Finds it not as satisfactory as *Seize the Day*, his best novel, or *The Adventures of Augie March*.

Clayton, John J. "Alienation and Masochism." Bloomington: Indiana UP, 1968. 2nd ed. 1979. Rpt. in *Saul Bellow*. Ed. Harold Bloom. Modern Critical Views. New York: Chelsea, 1986. 65–85.

Discusses the paradox of Bellow's personal despair and romantic idealism; his Jewish humanism and guilt; his self-hatred and despair. Details evidences of Bellow's despair creeping into his fiction. Concludes that Bellow, like his heroes, is "life-affirming, love-affirming, individual-affirming. But underneath the 'yea' is a deep, persuasive 'nay'—underneath belief in the individual and in the possibility of community is alienation, masochism, despair."

———. "Saul Bellow's *Seize the Day*: A Study in Mid-Life Transition." *Saul Bellow Journal* 5.1 (1986): 34–37.

Argues for a positive ending in the novel based on the study of Wilhelm as an infantile regressive, who while in the midst of a mid-life crisis, takes steps toward true maturity as he mourns the corpse (the casting off of his old self) and emerges from the experience more maturely and deeply connected with the world of human beings.

Cronin, Gloria L. "The Purgation of Twentieth Century Consciousness." *Interpretations: A Journal of Ideas, Analysis and Criticism* 16.1 (1986): 8–20.

Asserts that in *H* Bellow's primary intention was to demonstrate a hero ridding himself of all superfluous modernist ideas. The text is read as one of the century's major Anglo–American rejections of modernist ideas. Supporting arguments are drawn both from the text and Bellow's interviews and essays. Illustrates the thoroughness of Herzog's and therefore Bellow's analysis of exactly what the effects have been of the works of all the great modernist thinkers on the contemporary sense of the Self.

——. "Through a Glass Brightly: Dean Corde's Escape from History in *The Dean's December*." *Saul Bellow Journal* 5.1 (1986): 24–33.

Corde is seen as Bellow's tool for resolving the longstanding issue in Western Civilization between empirical and mystical modes of knowing. Corde becomes the pioneer who eschews the visions of society conferred by ordinary consciousness and who seeks to penetrate the *fantasmo imperium* where real facts are covered from human perception. Beyond that, he is also the fictional means by which Bellow and the reader may escape the reductive and nihilistic fabric of twentieth-century history to a corrected vision of that transcendental harmony both within the individual and throughout the larger creation, a harmony discernible only to the person of corrected vision, perceptual and emotional.

Fuchs, Daniel. "On *Him with His Foot in His Mouth and Other Stories*." *Saul Bellow Journal* 5.1 (1986): 3–15.

General review of several stories in the volume.

——. "Saul Bellow and the Example of Dostoevsky." Ed. Duane J. MacMillan. Toronto: U of Toronto P, 1979. 157–76. Originally delivered as a lecture at the second annual meeting of the Austrian American Studies Association, Schloss Leopoldskron, Salzburg, Oct. 1955; revised version rpt. in *Saul Bellow: Vision and Revision*. Durham, NC: Duke UP, 1984. 28–49; *Saul Bellow*. Ed. Harold Bloom. Modern Critical Views. New York: Chelsea, 1986. 211–33.

Denies that we can go on saying with Hemingway that all American literature comes from *Huckleberry Finn*. Much contemporary American literature comes from Flaubert and the Russians. Bellow is the leading exponent of the Russian way in American literature. Of particular note is the influence of Dostoevsky on Bellow. An erudite and major analysis.

Goldman, Liela H. "*The Dean's December*: A Companion Piece to *Mr. Sammler's Planet*." *Saul Bellow Journal* 5.2 (1986): 36–45.

Discusses the extent to which *DD* bears an affinity to *MSP*. Compares the two works in terms of global political concerns, the deaths of key characters, repressive urban environments, moral/ethical alienation, the sacredness that lies at the core of life, the value of the individual, mood, tone, and style.

——. "The Holocaust in the Novels of Saul Bellow." *Modern Language Studies* 16.1 (1986): 71–80.

Describes Bellow's statement on the subject of the Holocaust in terms of his analysis of the misguided Romantic origins of German culture, which in turn gave rise to the phenomenon of Nazism. Goldman sees Nazism as an attack on Western Humanism and characterizes Bellow's novelistic processes of thought as consistently Jewish in their defense of humanistic philosophy. Discusses miso-Germanism in terms of specific Bellow characters throughout the novels and in terms of Bellow's critique of German philosophers responsible for the intellectual basis of German Romanticism.

Guieu, Ives. "Le Machiavel et le mystique ou les deux avatars de heros de Saul Bellow." *Etudes Anglaises* 39.4 (1986): 444–50.

Hall, Joe. *"The Dean's December*: A Separate Account of a Separate Account." *Saul Bellow Journal* 5.2 (1986): 22–32.

Provides a defense and explanation of Bellow's experimentation with the seemingly plotless novel of reflection and philosophical thought. Describes Corde as a "satisfying artistic embodiment of the narrator's puzzling over his sense of ethical outrage; he finds his sources for judgment in the classical ethical tradition of Western Civilization, but he finds at the same time that this tradition and the account of the world which sustained it are dying."

Hollander, John. "Return to the Source." *Harper's* (Dec. 1976): 84–85. Rpt. as "To Jerusalem and Back." *Saul Bellow.* Ed. Harold Bloom. Modern Critical Views. New York: Chelsea, 1986. 97–100.

Describes the trip depicted in the book as an inward and backward, as well as an outward and onward, journey. Suggests that the book has as much to do with the diaspora Jew traveling to a lately marked-out center and home again to exile as it has to do with Israel itself. Describes the book as being as full of talk as encounter and of asking one central question about the survival of Israel. Discusses the "grotesque awkwardness" with which Bellow depicts the Israeli political experiment. Describes also the shadow of Russian literature and the history of the Middle East itself. Concludes that what gives the book unity is the author's fierce personality as referee. A major article.

Howe, Irving. "Odysseus Flat on His Back." *New Republic* 19 Sept. 1964: 21–26. Rpt. as "Herzog." *The Critic as Artist: Essays on Books 1920–1970.* Ed. Gilbert A. Harrison. New York: Liveright, 1972. 181–91; as "Down and Out in New

York and Chicago: Saul Bellow, Professor Herzog, and Mr. Sammler." *The Critical Point: On Literature and Culture.* Ed. Irving Howe. New York: Horizon, 1973. 121–36, and *Herzog: Text and Criticism.* Ed. Irving Howe. Viking Critical Library. New York: Viking, 1976. 391–400. Rpt. with original title in *Saul Bellow.* Ed. Harold Bloom. Modern Critical Views. New York: Chelsea, 1986. 45–51.

Praises Bellow as one of the most powerful minds among contemporary American writers and one "who best assimilates his intelligence to creative purpose." However, he has "become increasingly devoted to the idea of the novel as sheer spectacle." Howe sees *H* as Bellow's most remarkable and notably advanced novel in technique. Complains that instead of freeing us from the image of the sick self, we are still caught up with it in this novel. Howe sees the novel primarily as a remarkably animated performance combining both the despairing and the comic.

Hughes, Daniel J. "Reality and the Hero: *Lolita* and *Henderson the Rain King.*" *Modern Fiction Studies* 6.4 (1960–61): 345–64. Rpt. *Saul Bellow and the Critics.* Ed. Irving Malin. New York: New York UP, 1967. 69–91; *Saul Bellow.* Ed. Harold Bloom. Modern Critical Views. New York: Chelsea, 1986. 25–43.

Both novels read in conjunction throw light on the problems of the contemporary novelist and the much-heralded crisis in the novel. Both are novels about the quest for reality on the part of protagonists who completely fill the novels in which they appear but who are not satisfied with such a role. Hughes goes on to make a series of complex and enlightening comments on similarities and differences between the two novels.

Hynes, Joseph. "The Fading Figure in the Worn Carpet." *Arizona Quarterly* 42.3 (1986): 321–30.

Provides a general discussion of traditional moralists in the twentieth-century novelistic tradition which encompasses Bellow. Discusses Bellow's alienation of his old liberal readership through his detailed denunciation of a society which has produced a black underclass and the urban nightmare city, social evils these old sympathizers now do not want to hear about. To this extent he sees a remarkable affinity between Bellow and James.

Kaler, Anne K. "Use of the Journal/Diary Form in the Development of the Odyssean Myth in *Dangling Man*." *Saul Bellow Journal* 5.1 (1986): 16–23.

Argues that modern man has no exterior voice such as a gleeman or scop. The modern anti-hero has only his own voice which is not intended for public oral presentation but for private reading. This ancient and yet modern voice has been achieved through the journal voice in *DM* and functions to underscore his sung epic as he develops a modern version of the Odyssean myth in the novel.

Kernan, Alvin B. "Mighty Poets in their Misery Dead: The Death of the Poet in Saul Bellow's *Humboldt's Gift*." Alvin B. Kernan. Princeton: Princeton UP, 1982. 37–65. Abridged version rpt. in *Saul Bellow*. Ed. Harold Bloom. Modern Critical Views. New York: Chelsea, 1986. 161–77.

Spends considerable time tracing the historical evolution and devolution of the social role of the poet. Comments that in modern times poets within the works are depicted as dismembered and demystified, not by philosophic and psychological anxieties, but by historical and social events generating those anxieties. Sees *HG* as a novel in which literature as a social institution is subject for its continued validity to the situation in the larger society. *HG* offers insights into the nature of the social changes which are unmaking that grand image of the poet and his powers Petrarch constructed so long ago in Rome.

Kerner, David. "The Incomplete Dialectic of *Humboldt's Gift*." *Dalhousie Review* 62.1 (1982): 14–35. Rpt. in *Saul Bellow*. Ed. Harold Bloom. Modern Critical Views. New York: Chelsea, 1986. 161–77.

HG centers on the theme of spiritual rebirth and escape from mortality, as evidenced by Humboldt's escape from madness and spiritual return seven years later. This irrepressibility establishes the connections between the self and the divine powers, so that the reprieved Humboldt can claim we are "supernatural beings," but these divine powers are the "inner powers of nature," which "art manifests." Yet Bellow knows that salvationist art cannot wish away rationalism. Bellow shows us Humboldt's box and chains from the outside only, as when a showman presenting an escape artist is afraid to let us examine the arrangements too closely.

Knight, Karl F. "Bellow's 'Cousins': The Suspense of Playing It to the End." *Saul Bellow Journal* 5.2 (1986): 32-35.

The principal theme in Saul Bellow's "Cousins" is the effort to hold things together against the forces of dissolution. Ijah Brodsky, the protagonist, has an apocalyptic sense of the struggle, but avoids despair by working for continuity within his family, by being a responsive and responsible cousin. But the story suggests too that responsibility to the larger society may at times take precedence over loyalty to a particular cousin; indeed, the term "cousins" comes to mean the universal human family.

Marcus, Steven. "Reading the Illegible: Some Modern Representations of Urban Experience." *Southern Review* [Baton Rouge] 22.3 (1986): 443-64.

Examines the works of Bellow and Pynchon for evidence of their classical depictions of a modern conception of the city. Likens Bellow's Chicago to the Dublin of Joyce, the London of Dickens and the Paris of Balzac. Contains an extremely thorough treatment of each novel in turn. Perhaps the major treatment of the subject of Bellow's cityscapes.

Marotti, Maria Ornella. "Concealment and Revelation: The Binary Structure of *Seize the Day*." *Saul Bellow Journal* 5.2 (1986): 46-51.

Discusses the idea that though the novel is centered on a central character's facing a moment of deep crisis and self-discovery, the novella is organized through the principle of a shifting center

of consciousness which is functional to the deep structure of the
text, the underlying binary pattern of concealment and revelation.
In fact, not only is the reader allowed to penetrate the true emotional roots of the protagonist's personality through his thoughts,
delusions, and memories, but s/he can also see the impact of his
appearance on the world through his father's thoughts and the
narrator's grotesque descriptions of his discordant physical traits.

McCord, Phyllis Frus. " 'A Specter Viewed by a Specter':
     Autobiography in Biography." *Biography: An Interdisciplinary
     Quarterly* 9.3 (1986): 219–28.

Uses the example of Bellow's dissatisfaction with Mark Harris's
biographical attempts at depicting him for a general discussion
on the contemporary theory of biographical literature and the
disruption of the Harris biography on Bellow.

Morahg, Gilead. "The Art of Dr. Tamkin: Matter and Manner
     in *Seize the Day*." *Modern Fiction Studies* 25.1 (1979): 103–16.
     Rpt. in *Saul Bellow*. Ed. Harold Bloom. Modern Critical Views.
     New York: Chelsea, 1986. 147–59.

SD is problematic in that its intellectual values depend heavily
on the enigmatic character of Dr. Tamkin, who through seemingly
negative ideas communicates positive healing effects. Morahg
provides a good review of critical assessments of Tamkin. Tamkin,
like the literary artist, uses his imaginative vision to communicate
cogent visions of human reality. These are generally analogous
to a developing vision postulated in Bellow's later novels. Like
Bellow, he is dedicated to a cultural and spiritual mission he
believes can be carried out through his art. Morahg traces these
ideas in considerable detail throughout this and later novels.

Nilsen, Helge Normann. "A New Kind of Male–Female Rela-
     tionship: A Note on Saul Bellow's *The Dean's December*."
     International Fiction Review 13.2 (1986): 89–92.

Observes that in most of Bellow's novels "Bellow's heroes
have typically suffered from a phobic and paranoid reaction to

women and their expectations of love and emotional commitment. As a result they become isolated, lose contact with their children, and suffer from the guilt feelings that follow.'' In *DD* the male–female relationships show a remarkable improvement; Corde transcends the total ego absorption of the earlier male characters and allows himself to become domesticated. Nilsen provides a careful description of each of the relationships with women that Dean Corde establishes.

Ozik, Cynthia. "Farcical Combat in a Busy World." *New York Times Book Review* 20 May 1984: 3. Rpt. in *Saul Bellow*. Ed. Harold Bloom. Modern Critical Views. New York: Chelsea, 1986. 235–41.

Calls the volume *Him with His Foot in His Mouth* ''a concordance, a reprise, a summary, all the old themes and obsessions hauled up by a single tough rope.'' Praises the work further as a ''cumulative art concentrated, so to speak, in a vial.'' Sees the stories as the long-awaited personal decoding process for Bellow. Comments on each story and places Bellow in his twentieth-century American and international context. Major review essay to date.

Pugh, Scott. "Preemptive Defense of Narrative and the Designs of *The Deans's December.*" *Kyushu American Literature* 27 (1986): 87–95. Cited in *MLA Bibliography* (online).

Argues that Bellow employs a large range of devices aimed at preventing the reader from easy systematizing and categorizing of the author or his works. With regard to *DD* he claims that Corde is no more unable to accept his own conclusions and advice than the reader is. These distortions and evasions of style are even mirrored in the Dean's appearance, as well as in the opening paragraphs of the novel. Also, ''various everymen are variously posed and counterposed, thereby providing maximum resistance to evaluation.'' The collection abounds in ''models for misreading.'' Concludes that the novel provides a broad range of stances from which the world can be viewed—''business, bureaucracy, science, religion, humanism, communism''—but in their juxtapositions their respective distortions become glaring.

Shoham, Karen "SQL: Un modele pour une base de donnees lexicologiques." *Trauvaux de Linguistique Quantitative 35.* Geneva: Slatkine, 1986. 797–806. Papers from an international colloquium on Computers in Literary & Linguistic Research, University of Nice, June 5–8, 1985.

Warren, Robert Penn. "The Man with No Commitments." *New Republic* 2 Nov. 1953: 22–23. Rpt. in *Saul Bellow.* Ed. Harold Bloom. Modern Critical Views. New York: Chelsea, 1986. 9–12.

Sees *AM* as Bellow's most important novel to date. Identifies Augie as a "latter-day example of the Emersonian ideal Yankee who could do a little of this and a little of that." Criticizes Augie for having no commitments and for being a static character.

Weinstein, Mark. "Communication in *The Dean's December.*" *Saul Bellow Journal* 5.1 (1986): 63–74.

Sees the main subject of *DD* as that of communication on a variety of levels—personal, political, philosophical and societal. Especially explored is the subject of communication in both an open and a closed society. Argues that *DD* is a tightly organized novel when viewed from this perspective.

Yetman, Michael G. "Toward a Language Irresistible: Saul Bellow and the Romance of Poetry." *Papers on Language & Literature* 22.4 (1986): 429–47.

Asserts that *DD* presents a personal view of modern urban life as opposed to an official engineer's, sociologist's, anthropologist's or politician's view. *DD* represents "a dismissal 'with contempt,' of the non-poetic, objectivist contemporary social thought." Says Bellow has a " 'logocentric vision of language' as both creator and vehicle of personal vision" that assumes a symbiotic relationship between language and experience. Despite Derrida's deauthorizing of language while simultaneously denying its referential function, Bellow reminds us, "Some of the best imaginative writing today continues to implicitly assert the Coleridgean belief that language is a conduit between mind and reality, that words reflect and at the same time interpret, humanize, even 'save' through imagination the stuff of literal experience.'' ''With its romantic underpinnings, logocentrism is useful to an assessment of *DD*.'' Also provides a treatment of the political ideas contained in the novel.

Interview

Ignatieff, Michael. ''Our Valuation of Human Life Has Become Thinner.'' *The Listener* 13 March 1986: 18–19.

Reviews

Bertens, H. Rev. of *Fiction as Survival Strategy: A Comparative Study of the Major Works of Ernest Hemingway and Saul Bellow*, by Jan Bakker. *Dutch Quarterly Review of Anglo-American Letters* 16.1 (1986): 77–80.

Braham, Jeanne, Rev. of *Saul Bellow's Moral Vision: A Critical Study of the Jewish Experience*, by Liela H. Goldman. *Modern Fiction Studies* 31.4 (1986): 740–45.

———. Rev. of *On Bellow's Planet: Readings from the Dark Side*, by Jonathan Wilson. *Modern Fiction Studies* 32.4 (1986): 621–23.

Minot, S. Rev. of *Great Jewish Short Stories*, ed. Saul Bellow. *North American Review* 271.1 (1986): 76–80.

Newman, Judie. Rev. of *Saul Bellow: Vision and Revision*, by Daniel Fuchs. *Journal of American Studies* 20.2 (1986): 309–10.

O'Connell, Shaun. Rev. of *On Bellow's Planet: Readings from the Dark Side*, by Jonathan Wilson. *American Literature* 58.4 (1986): 663–64.

Rev. of *On Bellow's Planet: Readings from the Dark Side*, by Jonathan Wilson. *Choice* May 1986: 1395.

Rev. of *Him with His Foot in His Mouth and Other Stories*, by Saul Bellow. *KLIATT Young Adult Paperback Book Guide* Jan. 1986: 28.

Rev. of *Him with His Foot in His Mouth and Other Stories*, by Saul Bellow. *Observer* (London) 20 Jan. 1986: 23.

Rev. of *Him with His Foot in His Mouth and Other Stories*, by Saul Bellow. *Observer* (London) 23 Feb. 1986: 28.

Sakano, T. Rev of *Saul Bellow: Vision and Revision*, by Daniel Fuchs. *Studies in English Literature* [Tokyo] 63.1 (1986): 186–91.

Dissertations

Blustein, Bryna Lee. *Beyond the Stereotype: A Study of Representative Short Stories of Selected Contemporary Jewish American Female Writers* (Yezierska, Olsen, Paley, Darwin, Ozick). Diss. St. Louis University, 1986.

Traditionally, Jewish women have been placed in an inferior role. Such authors as Bernard Malamud, Saul Bellow, and Philip Roth, writing within the parameters of their genres, perpetuate the cultural image of the subordinate Jewish woman. In their short stories they present three negative stereotypes of the Jewish American woman: Malamud's first generation defeated "Yiddish Momma," Bellow's second generation domineering wife and mother, and Roth's third generation "Jewish American Princess." In the process of their storytelling, these male writers bypass the real nature and concerns of women. Not unexpectedly, contemporary Jewish American female short story writers have repudiated the notion that the Jewish American woman is reducible to a caricature. They have looked beyond the stereotype and given their female characters traits of individuality. This study depicts the developing literary voice of Jewish women and looks at the stories that women tell about themselves. Anzia Yezierska, who published two short story collections, *Children of Loneliness* and *Hungry Hearts* in the '20s, is the lone spokeswoman for the ambitious immigrant woman. Thirty years later, in her collection *Tell Me a Riddle*, Olsen depicts Everywoman who must helplessly subordinate herself to her family. The heroine of many of the short stories found in Grace Paley's *Enormous Changes at the Last Minute* and *The Little Disturbances of Man* is Faith Darwin, a Bohemian of the '60s. Ozick's extraordinary women, found primarily in *Leviation*, are strongly connected to Jewish myth and legend. Olsen, Paley, and Ozick have rigorously examined the Jewish American woman and found her to be a fully realized human being. By humanizing their characters, women writers have attempted to destroy the stereotype created by Jewish American male short story writers. This study, then, is not a rebuttal. This study looks at the literature that records, reflects, and affirms the possibilities of women's lives.

Fox, Francis Patrick. *Saul Bellow's City Fiction*. Diss. University of Pennsylvania, 1986.

The dissertation focuses on the challenge the city and city experience have posed to Bellow throughout his career. The dissertation begins by examining the works of Bellow's literary apprenticeship, *Dangling Man* and *The Victim*. It follows Bellow's first, self-conscious efforts to find his place as a city writer and intellectual in the tradition of modern urban fiction and to come to terms as a city man and Jew with the emerging cosmopolitan world of postwar America. The dissertation continues with an examination of *Augie March* and *Seize the Day*. It reveals Bellow forging his original voice as a city writer, while establishing the continuity of his development from a literary apprentice to a literary master. The dissertation then turns to *Henderson the Rain King*, Bellow's only major work without a dominant city setting. Examining Henderson's quest, the dissertation confirms Bellow's observation that he cannot "possibly separate my knowledge of life, such as it is, from the city" and his judgment that from *Henderson* he "dates being in fullest command of his powers."

The dissertation then attends to the success that meets Bellow's efforts in *Herzog* and *Sammler's Planet* to adapt his mature style to the demands of his own native ground. Here, Bellow realizes what had been his ambition, but not his accomplishment as a young writer, when he took as the subject of his art the challenge of the city which informs all later fiction. The dissertation concludes with a brief consideration of *Humboldt's Gift*. A compendium of the many uses Bellow has made of the city in his long career, *Humboldt's Gift* offers a fitting coda to a study of his accomplishment as a city writer. In Bellow's thinly veiled memoir of the progress of his generation of city Jews and city intellectuals from interlopers on the American scene to media celebrities and culture heroes, it finds a valediction for his generation's formative role in enacting and interpreting the public spectacles and private dramas of an America discovering itself as an irremediably urban world.

Tackach, James M. *The Huck Finn Hero in Modern American Fiction*. Diss. University of Rhode Island, 1986.

In creating Huck Finn, Mark Twain created an archetypal American hero, a character to whom American writers return again and again. This dissertation identifies the main characteristics of the "Huck Finn hero" created by Twain and recast in various settings and social milieus by modern American fiction writers. One hundred years after the publication of Twain's *Adventures of Huckleberry Finn*, American writers are still writing books featuring the Huck Finn hero. There is a group of modern novels whose heroes closely resemble Twain's Huck. Variations are many, but in its purest form this Huck Finn hero is a boy (or a young man), usually an orphan or a child missing a parent, who leaves home; has a violent clash with the "civilized" world; in a crucial moment—when he faces a difficult moral choice—rejects society's moral code in favor of his own impulsive, intuitive code of ethics; then "lights out for the territory," a final repudiation of American society. The modern works used in this study to demonstrate the persistence of the Huck Finn hero include major works of American fiction as well as "popular" novels; they span the modern literary era, and they are varied in setting: Ernest Hemingway's Nick Adams stories, William Faulkner's *The Bear* (and other Ike McCaslin stories), Saul Bellow's *The Adventures of Augie March*, Ralph Ellison's *Invisible Man*, Mark Harris's *The Southpaw*, Joseph Heller's *Catch-22*, Norman Mailer's *Why Are We in Vietnam?* and Dan Jenkins' *Semi-Tough*. The works are grouped and discussed in terms of setting. Chapter I defines the Huck Finn hero. Chapter II presents the Huck Finn hero on the battlefield; the Nick Adams stories and *Catch 22* are discussed in this chapter. Chapter III presents Huck on the ballfield, and *The Southpaw* and *Semi-Tough* are discussed there. Chapters IV and V present the Huck Finn hero in the city and the wilderness; Chapter IV discusses *Augie March* and *Invisible Man*, and Chapter V discusses *The Bear* and *Why Are We in Vietnam?* The conclusion, Chapter VI, analyzes the reasons for the persistence of the Huck Finn hero in American literary history.